Radioactivity in Life Sciences

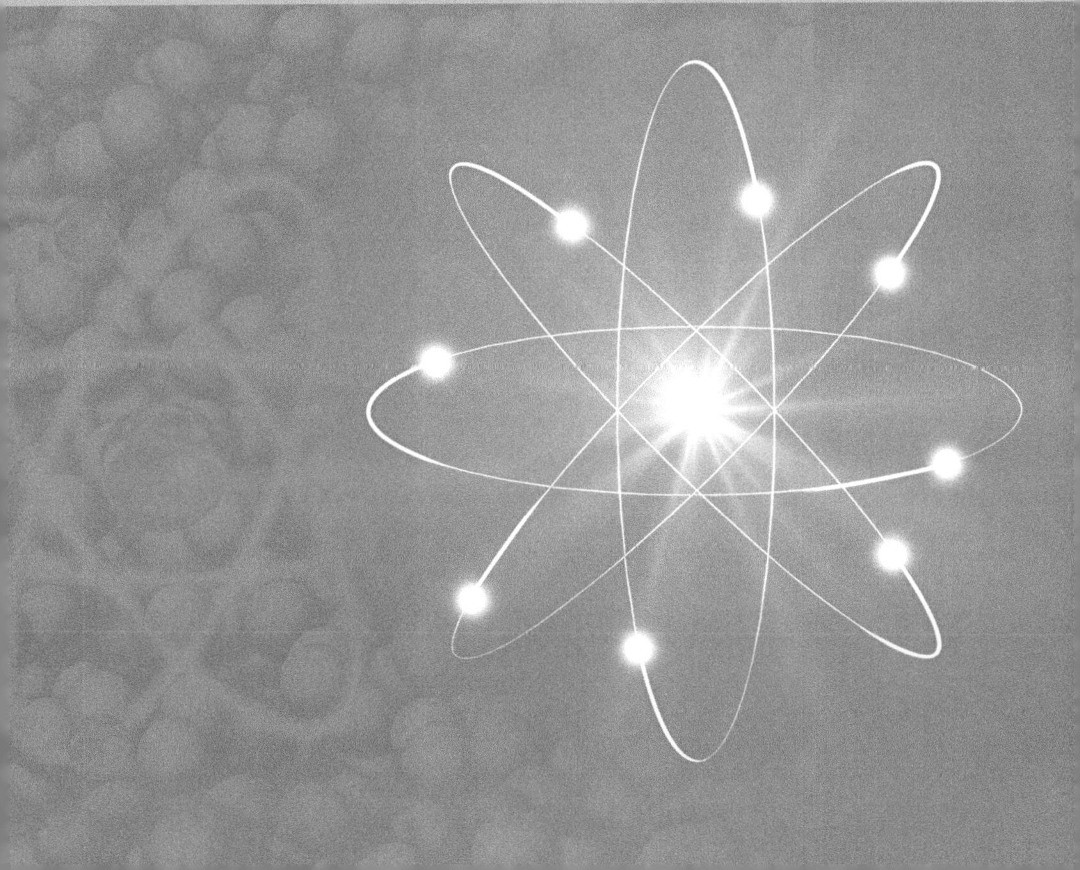

Radioactivity in Life Sciences

edited by
Maria Letizia Terranova

JENNY STANFORD
PUBLISHING

Published by

Jenny Stanford Publishing Pte. Ltd.
101 Thomson Road
#06-01, United Square
Singapore 307591

Email: editorial@jennystanford.com
Web: www.jennystanford.com

British Library Cataloguing-in-Publication Data
A catalogue record for this book is available from the British Library.

Radioactivity in Life Sciences

ISBN 978-981-5129-67-0 (Hardcover)
ISBN 978-1-003-63654-0 (eBook)

Contents

Preface

Two of the big challenges of the present times, namely reducing CO_2 emissions and achieving geopolitical energy independence, rely on the replacement of fossil fuels by other energy sources. The transition toward clean and affordable energy involves a mixed scenario that also includes power produced by nuclear technologies.

However, socio-scientific controversies about the risks arising from ionizing radiation not only make a tangible impact on the acceptance of nuclear power but also endanger the development of nuclear technologies in fields ranging from health care to agriculture and research.

Regardless of the position taken in this debate, one must recognize that in less than a century, the topic of radioactivity has shifted from great public appreciation to deep fear and from an extensive (often exaggerated) use to expressions of strong dissent.

A fundamental change of perspective about radioactivity started in 1956 when the US National Academy of Sciences published a study on the changes that were induced in the human genome by radiation. Later a study on the atomic bomb survivors suggested the relationship between radiation exposure and cancer cases. This was at the time of the Cold War, and a public opinion plagued by the threat of a nuclear attack extended the fear of ionizing radiation to civil nuclear facilities and medical procedures. In this context, the National Committee on Radiation Protection adopted a precautionary policy based on the linear no-threshold (LNT) principle. All the other countries accepted the NCRP recommendations and still represent a legacy issue with which present nuclear technologies have to deal.

The accidents that took place at Chernobyl and Fukushima certainly did not help to change the public perception or mitigate concerns about radioactivity and its effects on life. A generalized lack of scientific knowledge and, subsequently, the widespread misinformation acted as a sounding board that amplified concerns about safety hazards.

In this context, it was, therefore, thought important to create a rational image of radioactivity and to distinguish trustworthy notions/concepts from the background noise produced by a wide range of unchecked information sources.

The purpose of this book is to provide a clear description of the role played by radioactivity in the living world as well as of the implications of ionizing radiations in life sciences.

The book features nine chapters that provide, from a multidisciplinary perspective, an up-to-date look at the ongoing studies and elucidate with concrete examples the various aspects of ionizing radiation and their impact on biological systems.

Chapter 1 by Prof. Sutou starts with a description of natural and artificial radioactivity and goes on to highlight the existence of an efficient biological defense mechanism against damages produced by low-dose ionizing radiation in living organisms. Describing the relationship between ionizing radiations and life, the chapter introduces the issue of "radiation hormesis," a concept that extends to radioactivity the well-known "chemical hormesis," the biphasic dose-dependent response to drugs.

Among the several examples of radiation hormesis, this chapter presents data on lifespan and cancer cases of the Hiroshima and Nagasaki A-bomb survivors and people exposed to the Fukushima Daiichi nuclear power plant accident. The statistical analysis of such data is supplemented by considerations regarding natural radioactivity and consequent unavoidable exposures to internal and external radioactive sources. Some examples reported by Prof. Sutou anticipate the topic of background radiation and its impact on life, which are further developed in Chapter 6.

In addition, the chapter offers a brief historical overview of the radiation protection regulations established according to the controversial "LNT model," and discusses the validity of such a model and the current implications these LNT-based rules have on nuclear-based techniques that are employed in clinical practice.

The topic of natural radioactivity and its effects on the health of living organisms is put into a chronological context through a historical introduction to thermal springs by Dr. Rolls in Chapter 2. This chapter traces the scientific story of Bath, the United Kingdom's famous hot water spa—from the hypothesis advanced in the 18th century about an "aetherial essence" released by the hot waters to the studies performed in the 1920s that evidenced the presence of the radioactive gas Radon. It also describes the methods used in the past to administer this naturally occurring gas, the so-called "radium emanation," or prepare the many radon-based remedies proposed at the time to solve a series of diseases. Finally, the chapter discusses the change in attitudes of doctors and patients, from the initial enthusiasm for radioactivity-based therapies to the current unresolved controversy about the effects of low-dose radiation.

Chapter 3 focuses on the use of radiotherapy for benign disorders, linking the historical empirical protocols illustrated in Chapter 2 with the modern strategies employed nowadays to treat benign clinical conditions. A solid scientific background now enables us to clarify the physiopathological mechanisms underlying the more than 100 benign disorders that can be treated with radiotherapy. This chapter discusses the classification systems that are used to categorize the many different clinical conditions, either according to the anatomical sites involved or the main classes of disorders so far identified. Beyond explaining the radiobiological rationale, the authors review the indications of the benign conditions to be treated, mentioning the different protocols and RT schedules adopted in clinical practice by various institutions. The chapter also reports some selected clinical examples of benign diseases and discusses valid therapeutic options and alternatives to conventional medical adjuvants offered by recently developed radiotherapy techniques.

Chapter 4 showcases the significant promises of FLASH radiotherapy concerning the treatments of malignant diseases. This innovative technique uses an ultra-high dose rate of electrons produced by dedicated or modified linear accelerators (LINAC) to treat various cancer cases. The high-energy ionizing radiation at rates hundreds of times higher than that used in traditional radiotherapy allows administering the entire dose needed to eradicate the tumor in a single exposure. A further advantage of the FLASH approach is the reduction of the damage done to the exposed healthy tissues surrounding the tumor mass. The chapter describes the innovative configurations of the electron beams, the ongoing efforts to understand the radiobiological mechanisms responsible for FLASH effects, and the preclinical studies aimed at optimizing the therapeutical protocols. The translation of the challenging and ambitious FLASH strategy into a current clinical practice indeed requires defining a series of interdependent temporal parameters that include timing, dosage, and frequency of treatments.

The topic of the adaptive response to ionizing radiation, also outlined in other chapters, is specifically addressed in Chapter 5. In the chapter, Prof. Fornalsky explains the complex mechanism that allows cells exposed to low doses of ionizing radiation to develop an enhanced resistance to subsequent exposures to higher radiation doses. This unexpected adaptive response, first evidenced in studies conducted in the 1930s, indicates that for low levels of radioactivity, the relationship between radiation dose and biological effects could be much more complex than the proposed linear one. The implications of radio-adaptation in various fields, such as radiation protection, cancer-related studies, and clinical practice, have led to deep exploration of the phenomenon, aiming to confirm the experimental findings and to explain the observed non-targeted effects. The chapter presents the various mathematical and biophysical models proposed in the last two decades to integrate several aspects of the complex adaptive mechanism, from cell-type specific response to dose dependence and temporal dynamics. Also presented and discussed are the controversies, uncertainties, and limitations associated with the debated concept of radio-adaptation.

Chapter 6 deals with the research related to the growth of living organisms under low-radiation conditions. To avoid the natural background, which includes γ-rays, neutrons, muons, radon gas, and their daughter products originating in rocks and atmosphere, the reported experiments have all been conducted in deep underground laboratories (DUL). The authors present an updated review of the research conducted in the 1960s on single-celled organisms cultured in DUL as well as of the more recent ones on multicellular organisms. The chapter reports the most significant results obtained by research teams working in numerous underground laboratories spread all over the world. In this chapter, the authors analyze and debate the influence of low background radiation on cell proliferation and the biological response of various organisms. Overall, it is recognized that low levels of radiation can affect the cell metabolism and the organelles' function, increasing oxidative stress and reducing defense abilities. The findings reported in this chapter provide a scientific basis to understand the role that natural background radiation plays in life in a better way.

Moving from deep underground to space, Chapter 7 examines the additional challenges posed to astronauts' health by the out-of-earth environment, which is characterized by a high level of radioactivity. This chapter describes the several different countermeasures put into action to mitigate the threats associated with exposure to high radiation doses during long-term deep space missions. Beyond the engineering of specific materials and systems for advanced passive and active shielding, the reduction of health risks requires the development of a variety of medical actions. In this context, the chapter reviews the radioprotective pharmacologic agents to be administered before radiation exposure and the mitigators to be used after exposure to reduce the symptoms of radiation diseases. It also outlines biodefense practices, such as hibernation, immune system boosting, and adequate dietary regimes, and debates their efficiency in risk mitigation. In the chapter, again the topic of radio-adaptation, which is deeply addressed in Chapter 5, is discussed because the pre-flight screening of candidate astronauts involves an evaluation of their biological predispositions to radiation-adaptive response due to the fact that such biophysical phenomenon, associated with an individual genetic trait, could reduce the radiation-induced health risks.

Under the title "Social attitudes to ionizing radiation," Chapter 8 discusses the sources of social pressure that influence people's reactions to everything correlated with the topic "radioactivity." A generalized lack of scientific knowledge and the dominant misperception of the actual dangers produced even by low-dose exposure are the main factors that keep people away from forming their opinions, fueling undue anxiety about any kind of radioactive emissions.

To shed some light on the debated issue of ionizing radiation and to rationalize the concerns associated with their impact, Prof. Allison analyzes the different aspects of the interactions between radiation and living organisms separately.

His approach identifies three distinct aspects—physical, biological, and cultural—each characterized by its own time frame and by a specific logic. The first two are the initial physical damage and the subsequent biological response. The third aspect is the community attitude, consisting of personal and social reactions. The concise but clear elucidation of the radiation-induced physical and biological processes emphasizes a gap between the fear perceived by public opinion and the real dangers expected from exposures to low-dose ionizing radiation. As regards this last aspect, Chapter 8 explores the social response to radioactivity and nuclear technologies, relating the generalized anxieties provoked by them to the actual barrier between human perceptions of the outside world and the subjective self, a well-known mental mechanism responsible for the placebo and nocebo effects.

The book also expands to describe in Chapter 9 the issues associated with the management and transport of the radioactive sources used for civil applications. To ensure the safety of customers, the United Nations published the ADR regulation that details the criteria to be implemented for the safe transport of radioactive material. All the critical aspects of the transport of radioactive sources to specialized centers are taken into account in order to guarantee, beyond safety, the security of the operation. In the chapter, written by a recognized expert in radiation protection, the readers will find a short description of the main rules that regulate the procedures of the critical transport phase, from the choice of the ideal container to proper signaling.

The vision behind this editorial initiative is not to present an exhaustive review of all the aspects of ionizing radiation but to bridge boundaries between different scientific areas related to the common topic of radioactivity in life science. This selected collection of contributions from high-level authors has been conceived to give an opportunity to those wishing to enter this generally not familiar and often overlooked field of study and to connect the legacy of the past to the current debated scenario as well as future exciting perspectives.

Maria Letizia Terranova

January 2025

Chapter 1

Radiation and Chemical Hormesis: Low-Dose, Essential; Mid-Dose, Beneficial; High-Dose, Hazardous

Shizuyo Sutou
Shujitsu University, 1-6-1 Nishigawara, Naka-ku, Okayama-shi, Okayama 703-8516, Japan
sutou@shujitsu.jp

1.1 Introduction

Radiation was significantly intense at the dawn of life. Even today, we are consistently exposed to radiation, albeit at levels reduced to roughly one-fifth of its original potency, amounting to about 20,000 hits per second. It is worth noting that all foods and living organisms are naturally radioactive. Certain bacteria rely on radiation as their sole energy source. Additionally, numerous microorganisms on the ocean floor utilize H_2 generated through water radiolysis. Living organisms cannot survive well when shielded from ionizing radiation (IR), underscoring the indispensability of low-dose IR for

Radioactivity in Life Sciences
Edited by Maria Letizia Terranova

ISBN 978-981-5129-67-0 (Hardcover), 978-1-003-63654-0 (eBook)
www.jennystanford.com

life. A growing body of evidence supports hormesis, a phenomenon beneficial at mid-doses but hazardous at high-doses. The primary impact of IR on living organisms lies in the production of reactive oxygen species (ROSs), which serve as signaling agents. ROSs are chemical substances that undergo processing alongside other compounds within common metabolic systems. Substances supporting our lives also demonstrate hormetic responses. Currently, IR is regulated under the "linear no-threshold model (LNT)," which assumes that even the slightest radiation exposure carries an infinite risk. This model is also applied to carcinogens and mutagens. Our experimental investigations into the effects of mutagens have revealed a hormetic dose-response relationship. The validity of LNT is questionable, given our robust biological defense mechanisms such as DNA repair mechanisms, apoptosis, and immune responses. In the aftermath of the Fukushima Daiichi nuclear power plant accident, forced evacuations were carried out based on LNT, ostensibly to protect lives. However, in reality, not a single fatality resulted directly from radiation exposure. Unfortunately, the evacuation efforts led to over 2,000 casualties. This serves as a stark illustration of one of the darker aspects of LNT.

Following the Fukushima Daiichi Nuclear Power Plant (FDNPP) accident in 2011, a mandatory evacuation was implemented based on the LNT. In July, I volunteered to monitor radiation contamination among temporal returnees. At the same time, radiation contamination was measured at various locations. The highest value was 6,000 cpm, which scared me to think that my cancer risk might be increased, so I looked into the biological effects of radiation. As a result, we are exposed to approximately 20,000 hits per second internally and externally. The 6000 cpm is 100 cps, so I was very relieved to find that the extra 100 hits added to the 20,000 hits had little effect. Furthermore, I learned that there is a lot of data supporting radiation hormesis. In fact, when the lifespan and cancer risk of Hiroshima and Nagasaki A-bomb survivors were investigated, I found that they lived longer and had a lower cancer risk. For these reasons, the LNT that ionizing radiation (IR) is infinitely hazardous has been proven wrong. LNT is also applied to carcinogens and mutagens, and we conducted experiments on chemical hormesis using several mutagens and confirmed the occurrence of hormesis. In this paper, I show that LNT is false, radiation is essential and beneficial depending on doses, and the application of LNT to carcinogens and mutagens is false. Based on the LNT, I also point out that trying to protect people from harmless doses of radiation that can be extremely harmful.

1.2 Particle Beams and Radiation

1.2.1 Particle Beams

Radiation includes particle beams and electromagnetic waves. The main particle beams are α-rays, β-rays, and neutron beams. α-rays consist of the helium nucleus (two protons and two neutrons). α-rays have a strong ionizing ability, but their flight distance is short, about 30–40 μm in living organisms, i.e., the distance of 1–2 cells. Also, α-rays are bulky, so they can be blocked with a single piece of paper. The skin protects against external α-ray exposure.

β-rays are electron beams. In FDNPP, β-rays were mainly released from I-131, Cs-134, and Cs-137 (I-131 and Cs-137 also emit γ-rays). I-131 has a half-life of 8 days, so it decayed rapidly. The flight distance of β-rays derived from Cs-134 and Cs-137 is about 2 mm or less in the body. β-rays can be shielded by aluminum with a thickness of about 1 mm. Most of the radiation from the outside can be blocked by the skin. Fortunately, the skin is one of the least sensitive tissues to IR.

Neutrons are not formed in the normal decay series of U-235 and U-238. When fuel undergoes nuclear fission in a nuclear reactor or an A-bomb, 2–3 neutrons are released per fission. If the concentration of nuclear fuel is high, these neutrons collide with neighboring nuclei, causing a chain reaction that is used for nuclear power generation. Since neutrons are uncharged, they travel longer distances.

1.2.2 Electromagnetic Waves

Electromagnetic waves consist of a series of continuous wavelengths, and are roughly divided into radio waves, infrared rays, visible light, ultraviolet rays, X-rays, and γ-rays (Fig. 1.1). The shorter the wavelength, the stronger the energy. Depending on the wavelength, radio waves are used for radio-controlled clocks, radio broadcasts, FM broadcasts, televisions, microwave ovens, mobile phones, etc.

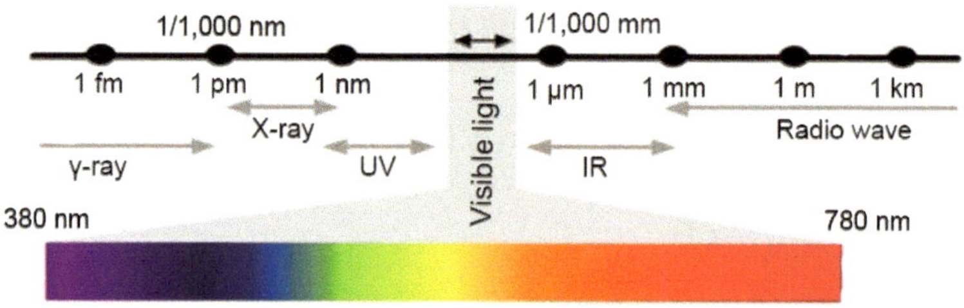

Figure 1.1 Types of electromagnetic waves. Electromagnetic waves consist of a series of wavelengths; but for convenience, they are named according to their wavelengths. The shorter the wavelength, the stronger the energy. The wavelength of visible light is 380–780 nm.

Infrared light is often used at airports to detect people with a fever. The powerful infrared rays from the A-bomb can instantly burn people to death. It causes the skin of survivors to swell and leave hypertrophic scars (keloids).

Since chlorophyll in plants uses blue and red lights for photosynthesis, green light is left behind and plants look green. Retinal cells in our eyes have proteins called opsins that can sense red, green, and blue wavelengths. Opsin combines with a chromophore called retinal to detect color. Retinal is made from vitamin A.

Adequate UV exposure is indispensable for vitamin D synthesis, while strong UV damages DNA. However, we have excellent repair mechanisms for DNA damage. When the amount of UV is large, we make melanin pigments and try to protect against injury caused by UV; but when the amount of UV is too much, the risk of skin cancer increases. The risk of developing malignant melanoma is 1–2 per 100,000 Japanese, while it reaches around 20 for white-skinned Westerners. Most of the UV rays from the Sun are absorbed by the ozone layer; but when the ozone hole is formed, the UV rays come directly to the ground, increasing the risk of skin cancer.

X-rays and γ-rays, which have shorter wavelengths than UV, have strong penetrating power and the ability to ionize molecules, so they are called ionizing radiation (IR). Ionization is to separate electrons from molecules. Therefore, the effects of X-rays and γ-rays are the same as those of particle beams. Since our bodies consist of approximately 70% water, electrons are knocked away from water molecules. As a result, reactive oxygen species (ROSs) are formed (Fig. 1.2). ROSs react with various biomolecules, including DNA, and affect living organisms. Macrophages and neutrophils phagocytize bacteria and other pathogens. ROSs such as superoxide anion (O_2^-) and hydrogen peroxide (H_2O_2) by the process of oxidative burst are released rapidly to kill them.

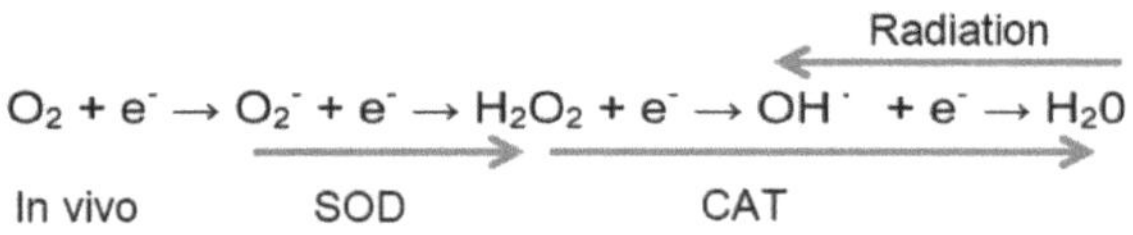

Figure 1.2 Formation of ROSs by ionizing radiation and elimination of these by enzymatic reactions in vivo. O_2^-, H_2O_2, and $OH^{\cdot}$ are ROSs. SOD indicates superoxide dismutase and CAT indicates catalase.

1.3 Radiation Is Ubiquitous

1.3.1 Relationship Between IR and Life

The relationship between IR and life is briefly shown (Fig. 1.3). Living organisms have been continuously exposed to IR and ingested radionuclides throughout their evolutionary history of 4 billion years (By). All living organisms are radioactive. Low-dose IR is essential for life. Some bacteria live using radiation as their sole energy source. A large number of microorganisms live on the radiolysis product H_2 as an energy source. IR generates ROSs, which are used as signaling agents by living organisms. Mid-dose IR is beneficial because it stimulates biological activities. Considering these, LNT—radiation is hazardous no matter how small the amount is—is invalid.

1.3.2 Radionuclides Are Abundant Around Us

Radionuclides are abundant in our surroundings (Table 1.1). Primary natural radionuclides with long half-lives have existed since the Earth's birth 4.6 By ago. The absorption dose unit Gy* is defined as 1 joule of radiation energy absorbed per kilogram of matter, meaning that the radiation ultimately produces heat. In fact, half of the Earth's heat is provided by the radioactive decay of radionuclides [2]. Although secondary natural radionuclides, which are daughters of primary radionuclides, have short half-lives, they are continuously produced. H-3 and C-14 are constantly generated in the air due to cosmic rays and are taken into living organisms. A typical artificial radionuclide is F-18, which is used for PET diagnosis.

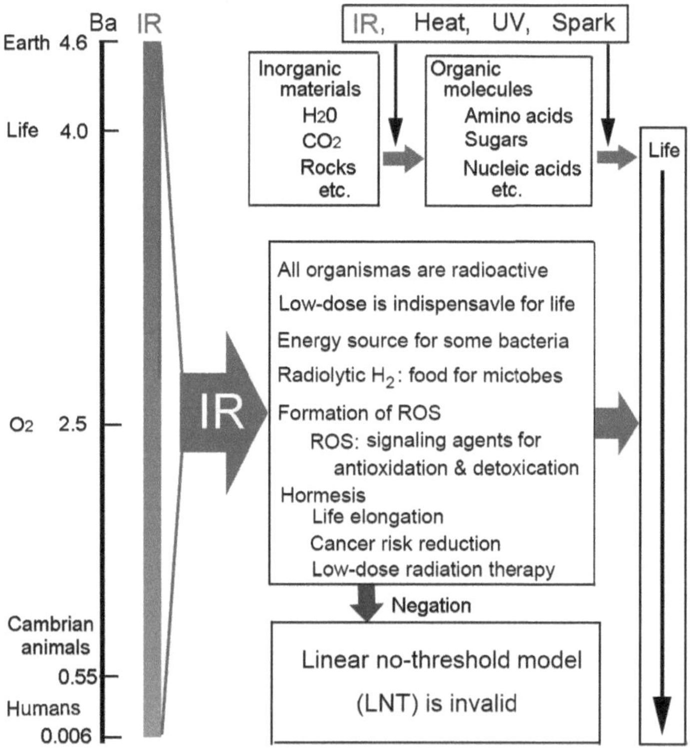

Figure 1.3 Relationship between ionizing radiation (IR) and life [1].

*To estimate human risk, the Sv unit is introduced; its use is limited to humans only. SV = Gy × radiation weighting factor × tissue weighting factor. These two factors are artificially determined, and the use of Gy is more scientific. Sv is used in this chapter as found in the source material, but it would not be a significant error to equate Sv with Gy in this context.

Table 1.1 Some examples of radionuclides around us

Primary natural radionuclides (present from the origin of the Earth)		
K-40	(Tτ: 1.25 By)	[Our body component]
U-235	(Tτ: 0.704 By)	[Parent isotope of the actinium series]
U-238	(Tτ: 4.46 By)	[Parent isotope of the uranium series]
Secondary natural radionuclides (daughters of primary natural radionuclides)		
Rn-222	(Tτ: 3.82 d)	[Daughter of U-238]
Induced radionuclides (generated continuously in the atmosphere by cosmic rays)		
Tritium	(Tτ: 12.3 y)	[By-product of nuclear power plants]
C-14	(Tτ: 5,730 y)	[Our body component]
Artificial radionuclides (produced with cyclotrons)		
F-18	(Tτ: 110 m)	[Used for PET diagnosis]

[Tτ: half-life; By: billion years; y: years; d: days; m: minutes]

1.3.3 All Foods and Living Organisms Are Radioactive

Table 1.2 shows the K-40 content in some Japanese foods. Although the content varies, all foods are radioactive. Similarly, all living organisms are radioactive.

Table 1.2 K-40 contents in Japanese foods (Bq/kg)

Food	K-40	Food	K-40
Beer	11	Spinach	192
Rice	33	Raw seaweed	226
Bread	29	Potato tips	370
Milk	52	Tea	851
Fish	133	Dried shiitake mushroom	666
Beef	115	Dried kelp	2,331

Source: The Nuclear Safety Research Association. Research on radiation data in living environment, Tokyo, 1983 [in Japanese].

1.3.4 We Receive 20,000 Hits per Second Internally and Externally

The content of K-40 in food is shown in Table 1.2, but we also ingest C-14, Po-210, and others. The subtotal 0.99 mSv/y of Japanese oral exposure dose is converted to 8,400 Bq (Table 1.3). Applying this ratio to the total exposure dose of Japanese people (2.1 mSv/y) yields 17,818 Bq. Similarly, the global average exposure dose is estimated to be 20,363 Bq. These Bq values are not always reasonable. For example, X-rays and γ-rays cannot be converted into Bq in principle. This figure (20,000 hits per second), however, provides a rough estimate of usual radiation exposure.

Table 1.3 Internal and external exposure doses of natural radiation

	Radiation source	**Effective dose (mSv/y)[a]**	**Bq[b]**
	C-14	0.01	2,590
Internal exposure	K-40	0.18	4,620
(Oral intake)	Rb-87	0.04	520
	Po-210, etc.	0.8	670
Subtotal		**0.99**	**8,400**
Internal exposure	Rn-222	0.37	
(Inhalation)	Thoron (Rn-220)	0.09	
	Smoking (Pb-210, Po-210, etc.)	0.006	
Subtotal		**0.476**	
External exposure	Cosmic rays	0.3	
	Radiation from the Earth	0.33	
Subtotal		**0.63**	
Japanese total		**2.1**	**17,818[c]**
US total		**3.11**	**26,387[c]**
Global average		**2.4**	**20,363[c]**

[a]The Nuclear Safety Research Association. New edition: Radiation in the living environment (Calculation of National Doses), Tokyo, 2011 [in Japanese].

[b]ibid., Research on radiation data in living environment, Tokyo, 1983 [in Japanese].

[c]The doses (Bq) were calculated proportionally using a conversion equation: 0.99 mSv/y are equal to 8,400 Bq.

1.3.5 Natural and Artificial Radiation

The average natural radiation in the world is 2.4 mGy/y. Still, there are high background radiation areas (HBRA) such as Ramsar in Iran (maximum 260 mGy), Kerala in India (35 Gy), and Guarapari in Brazil (35 Gy). I have seen many reports that there are no health hazards in HBRA.

Although above-ground nuclear tests were prohibited in 1963, underground tests continued, with a total of more than 2,500 nuclear tests being conducted. There are also approximately 450 nuclear power plants in operation around the world. However, the degree of global contamination caused by these is insignificant compared to natural radiation (Fig. 1.4). More attention is paid to medical exposure. However, the doses are not large enough to cause health problems. The contributions made through diagnosis and treatment are far more important.

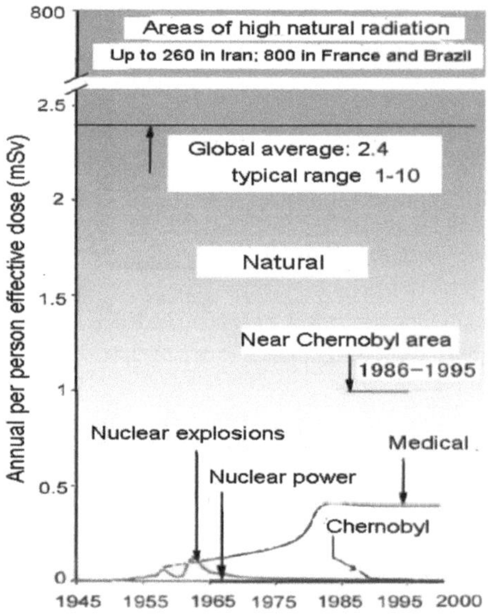

Figure 1.4 Comparison of natural radiation and artificial radiation [3].

1.4 Hormesis vs. LNT

Radiation is regulated by LNT. LNT tries to keep people as far away from radiation as possible because radiation is infinitely hazardous, and recommends the principle of "As Low As Reasonably Achievable (ALARA)." However, living organisms show an adaptive response called hormesis to tolerable stimuli, getting activated and energetic. In fact, experimental data show that dose-response curves are S-shaped, J-shaped, or reverse U-shaped, depending on experimental systems, and are never straight lines. Figure 1.5 shows that LNT and hormesis are incompatible with each other. The negative effects of LNT's ALARA precautionary principle are clearly demonstrated in the FDNPP accident, which forced unnecessary evacuations and resulted in more than 2,000 casualties.

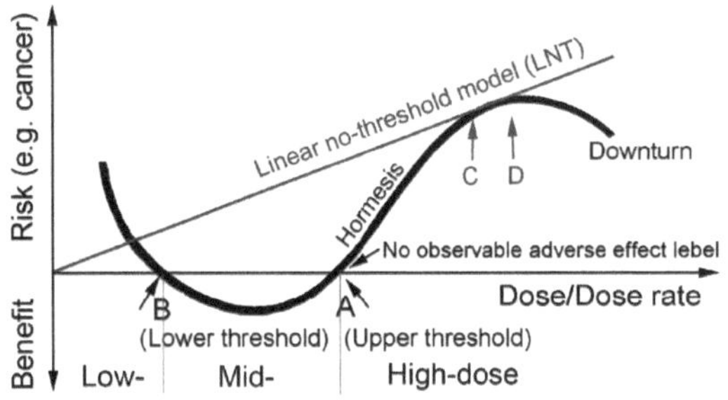

Figure 1.5 Schematic illustration of hormesis vs LNT [1]. The slanted S-shaped curve indicates the hormesis dose-response and the upward straight line from left to right indicates the LNT dose-response. If the dose is too high, the reaction is downturned. The hormesis curve intersects the x-axis at two points: A and B. Point A is the no observable adverse effect level (NOAEL), which is the so-called threshold. Point B is the lowest beneficial dose/dose rate, and between points A and B is the hormesis range. Doses below point B are the essential dose range. Points C and D of the LNT straight line show a pseudo-straight line in a hormetic response.

1.5 Not Scientific but Political Introduction of LNT

1.5.1 Strong Ties Between H. Muller and the Rockefeller Foundation

In 1914, Standard Oil established the Rockefeller Foundation (RF). One of its objectives was the "improvement of human welfare and education." RF must have focused on eugenics as a way to achieve human welfare. Eugenic ideology is the idea of protecting and nurturing the genes of those with superior physical and mental abilities, and conversely eliminating the genes of those with inferior abilities, thereby creating a superior society and human race.

In 1913, T. Morgan of Columbia University created a chromosome map using *Drosophila*. One of Morgan's students was H. Muller. He believed that humans should use genetics to control their evolution. Muller wrote that the future of mankind should not be left to "the free love of men and women." He was also the advocate of sperm banks. It is likely that RF resonated with Muller's eugenic ideas from the very beginning and welcomed him as its brain. Anyway, RF continued to support him until his death.

1.5.2 Muller's Controversial Science Paper

In 1927, H. Muller published a historic paper positing that X-rays induce mutations [4]. This seminal work later earned him the Nobel Prize. However, this paper is problematic, lacking essential elements such as methods, results, or references. Why was such a faulty paper published? At that time, the Science journal was privately owned by Columbia professor Cattell [5]. It appears that Muller negotiated well with Cattell and was able to publish the paper without peer review [6]. To secure the Nobel Prize, Muller had to lead the way.

In 1930, Muller introduced the proportionality rule [7], utilizing data from Oliver's studies [8]. This idea is the same as LNT that mutations occur in proportion to doses, and he continued to advocate LNT throughout his lifetime, disregarding conflicting scientific data.

1.5.3 Dishonesty in Muller's Nobel Prize Lecture

In 1942, the Manhattan Project was underway, dedicated not only to the production of A-bombs but also to the elucidation of the biological effects of radiation. While Stern of Stanford University led the *Drosophila* research, Muller was also engaged as a paid consultant and played a pivotal role in the research. In 1945, A-bombs were dropped on Hiroshima and Nagasaki, and people became concerned about the effects of radiation. In 1946, Muller was honored with the Nobel Prize. It is believed that the support from RF was significant.

During his Nobel Prize Lecture, Muller asserted that there is no threshold for the genetic effects of radiation [9]. However, it turned out that before the award lecture, he had obtained experimental data indicating the presence of a threshold. In an experiment using *Drosophila*, Caspari's data, which exhibited a notably high negative control value, indicated the existence of a threshold, while Uphoff's data, which displayed a low control value, suggested the absence of such a threshold [10]. Muller attributed the elevated values in Caspari's negative control to sampling errors and ultimately rejected the experienced Caspari's data in favor of the findings from master's student Uphoff. It is worth noting that the negative control values reported by Caspari were in close proximity to Muller's values, whereas Uphoff's control values were abnormally low. Calabrese accuses Muller of misrepresenting the experimental data [11].

1.5.4 Central Role of Muller and RF in the LNT Recommendation

In 1953, President Eisenhower gave a speech titled "Atoms for Peace" at the United Nations, opening nuclear power, which had previously been monopolized by government and military entities, to the private sector. In response, in 1954, the US National Academy of Sciences (NAS) chairman and RF director D. Bronk established the Committee on Biological Effects of Atomic Radiation (BEAR I) within the NAS. Sixteen members were appointed, but Muller was the central figure. W. Weaver, a board member of the RF and allocator of research funds, was selected as chair. LNT was recommended in 1956 without any proper discussion [12]. The significance of LNT is as follows: (1) The 500 mGy/y tolerable dose since 1934 has been drastically changed to "no threshold," meaning that radiation is infinitely genetically harmful. (2) It became the basis for the fallacious hypothesis that radiation induces cancer according to LNT. (3) The Environmental Protection Agency (EPA) has fallaciously decided that the carcinogenicity of carcinogens aligns with LNT. (4) It is still the basis of radiation regulations today.

The following are the problems with LNT: (1) The LNT paper has no author, and it is unclear who is responsible. (2) RF-funded NAS and several BEAR I committee members, constituting a contemporary conflict of interest. (3) The children of Hiroshima and Nagasaki A-bomb survivors showed that there are no genetic effects [13]. Neel's argument that people's matters should be based on people's data was rejected at Muller's insistence. (4) Among the predicted values of genetic effects submitted by the nine members of BEAR I, the three lowest data were arbitrarily discarded, and manipulations were made to create an impression of uniform high values. This can be called a fabrication. (5) Initially, J. Cuttler and later E. Calabrese petitioned M. McNutt, the editor-in-chief of Science at the time, to retract the LNT paper, but she declined [14]. (6) It was later discovered that the LNT paper was written by a magazine reporter and that the manuscript had not been circulated to the BEAR I committee members [15]. Based on this, Calabrese and others once again implored McNutt, who had moved from her editor-in-chief of Science to chair of NAS, the first female chair, to retract the LNT paper, but she refused again.

1.5.5 NAS's Error Again Regarding LNT

In 2006, NAS used data from Hiroshima and Nagasaki to propose that radiation-induced cancer risk follows LNT [16]. The main drawbacks are as follows: (1) Although both leukemia and solid cancers are purported to best fit the linear-quadratic dose-response relationship, NAS claims that solid cancers follow LNT because there is no statistically significant difference between the linear line and the linear-quadratic curve. (2) By limiting the upper limit of exposure dose to 2 Sv, downtown by higher doses is hidden. (3) Individuals who entered Hiroshima and Nagasaki after the A-bombing (NIC: not-in-the-city) are used as the negative control as zero exposure. However, they had been exposed to a considerable amount of residual radiation. Indeed, both threshold and hormesis can be observed in analysis using the Bayesian method, which does not require the use of negative controls [17]. (4) Neglecting residual radiation leads to an underestimation of radiation doses, consequently causing cancer risks to be overestimated. Including these, Sutou pointed out eight shortcomings of the NAS hypothesis [18]. As discussed later, it has been shown that, on average, A-bomb survivors lived longer and had a reduced cancer risk [19].

1.5.6 Unveiling the Dark Side of LNT Through FDNPP Accident

The International Commission on Radiological Protection (ICRP) places the LNT at the core of radiation prevention [20]. The FDNPP accident in March 2011 necessitated the evacuation of residents within a 20 km radius of the reactor, resulting in 2,337 disaster-associated deaths (Table 1.4). In Iwate and Miyagi, 470 (10.05%) and 931 (9.75%) deaths, respectively, were certified as disaster-associated, but these were not radiation-associated. When we apply the average proportion of disaster-associated deaths observed in Iwate and Miyagi (9.91%) to 1,614 Fukushima deaths, radiation-associated deaths would be 2,177, illustrating the victims of enforced evacuation as per the LNT (Table 1.4).

Table 1.4 Disasters- and nuclear accident-associated deaths from the Great East Japan Earthquake (The Reconstruction Agency, as of March 31, 2023)

Prefecture	**Deaths**	**Missing**	**Disaster-associated deaths (% of deaths)**	**Nuclear accident-associated deaths**
Iwate	4,675	1,110	470 (10.05%)	0
Miyagi	9,544	1,213	931 (9.75%)	0
Fukushima	1,614	196	2,337 (9.91% = 160*)	2,337 – 160 = 2,177*
Others	67	4	56	
Subtotal	15,900	2,523	3,794	
Total	**22,217**			

*Calculated by the author.

1.6 Radiation Hormesis

1.6.1 Bacteria "Eating" Ionizing Radiation (IR)

Desulforudis audaxviator bacterium lives in a 2.8 km deep gold mine in South Africa [21]. These are chemoautotrophic thermophiles that use the radiation energy of U-238 to obtain the basic ingredients of life from surrounding rocks. Similar bacteria were also found in a 2 km deep aquifer in eastern Siberia [22].

1.6.2 Microorganisms Thrive Deep Underground with the Support of IR

Many microorganisms live on the ocean floor, feeding on organic matter embedded in sediments or precipitated from the ocean. Beneath the sediments, basalt appears, followed by gabbro. These rock layers have pores and cracks through which seawater can seep. Biofilms form along these cracks. The total number of cells within the biofilm, consisting mainly of bacteria and archaea, is estimated to be 1.2×10^{30} cells [23]. Microbial cell density in subseafloor basalt can exceed 10^{10} cells/cm^3 [24]. The prosperity of life deep underground is supported by IR. Recent studies have shown that the radiolysis of water continuously produces H_2, which is the main electron donor (food) for microorganisms in continental aquifers several km below the earth's surface [25]. The deeper microorganisms live, the more they depend on radiolytic H_2, specially produced in rock formations.

1.6.3 Low-Dose Radiation (LDR) Is Essential: Shielding Experiment with Lead Bricks

In an experiment in which the protozoan *Tetrahymena* was irradiated with γ-rays, its proliferation was inhibited when it was shielded with lead bricks, and its proliferation was promoted when it was not shielded [26]. Similar findings were observed with cyanobacterium *Synechococcus lividus* [27]. In addition to these microorganisms, the growth or viability of the following organisms was also hindered by radiation shielding: *Mastigocladus laminosus* (alga), *Hordeum bonus* (barley), and *Artemia salina* (brine shrimp) [28].

1.6.4 LDR Is Essential: Deep Underground Experiments

Italy's Gran Sasso National Laboratory (LNGS) is situated beneath approximately 1,300 m of bedrock, creating an environment characterized by low background radiation levels. When *Saccharomyces cerevisiae* (yeast) was cultured and exposed to methyl methanesulfonate, a mutagen, it led to an increased mutation rate [29]. Similarly, Chinese hamster V79 cells exposed to γ-rays exhibited elevated mutation rates [30]. According to LNT, mutation rates should decrease in low-radiation environments.

The Waste Isolation Pilot Plant (WIPP) in Carlsbad, New Mexico, is positioned 650 m below the surface. When *Deinococcus radiodurans*, a radioresistant Gram-positive bacterium, was cultured there, its growth was significantly inhibited [31]. Transcription analyses indicated that background radiation is essential for normal growth [32]. Furthermore, the growth of V79 cells was similarly delayed when cultured in the WIPP environment [33].

1.6.5 LDR Is Essential: K-40 Deficiency Experiments

Of the 20,000 radiation hits, we receive every second, approximately 4,600 are attributed to K-40 (Table 1.3). Luckey investigated the effects of the lack of K-40 on organismal growth [28]. *Escherichia coli* (bacteria), *Tetrahymena pyriformis* (protozoa), mice, and rats showed significant growth retardation. Muckerheide [34] reported that mice fed a diet lacking K-40 showed reduced growth, but supplying K-40 restored growth. This result was not allowed for publication, because it was inconsistent with LNT.

1.6.6 Typical Data Demonstrating Hormesis

Radiation hormesis is prevalent in living organisms, and some illustrative examples are shown (Fig. 1.6). γ-Irradiation of *Tetrahymena* showed hormetic effects (Fig. 1.6A). The mutation rate of *Drosophila melanogaster* irradiated with X-rays showed a J-shaped dose-response curve, a hallmark of hormesis (Fig. 1.6B). The lifespan of mice irradiated with γ-rays for life increased at lower dose rates but decreased at higher dose rates (Fig. 1.6C). Given that, background radiation is 2.4 mGy/y, 1 to 10 mGy/d corresponds to 132 to 1,320 times background. When the relationship between radon levels and lung cancer incidence was investigated, the dose-response curve showed an inverse relationship and completely negated LNT (Fig. 1.6D). Some radon levels appear to be protective against lung cancer.

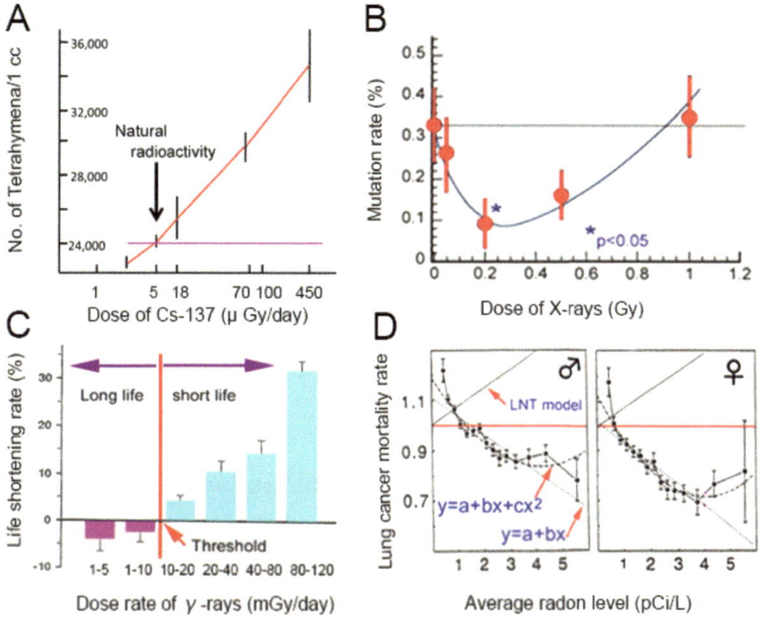

Figure 1.6 A typical example of radiation hormesis. (A) Growth inhibition and stimulation of *Tetrahymena* by gamma rays from Cs-137 [26]. (B) Mutation rate of *Drosophila melanogaster* irradiated with X-rays [35]. (C) The lifespan of mice irradiated with γ-rays for life [36]. (D) Relationship between radon levels and lung cancer incidence in 1,601 counties covering over 90% of the United States [37].

1.7 Hormesis in A-Bomb Survivors

1.7.1 Dropping of the A-Bomb on Hiroshima and Black Rain

On August 6, 1945, an A-bomb was dropped on Hiroshima. The energy consisted of 50% blast, 35% heat, and 15% radiation (Fig. 1.7A). Most people within a 1 km radius of the epicenter should die instantly from the blast and heat (Fig. 1.7B). The dose estimate was based only on the initial radiation (5%) and the residual radiation (10%) was ignored, resulting in an underestimate of the dose by approximately two times. Most of the residual radiation was from fallout that fell on the ground from black rain, so a wide area of Hiroshima City was contaminated (Fig. 1.7C).

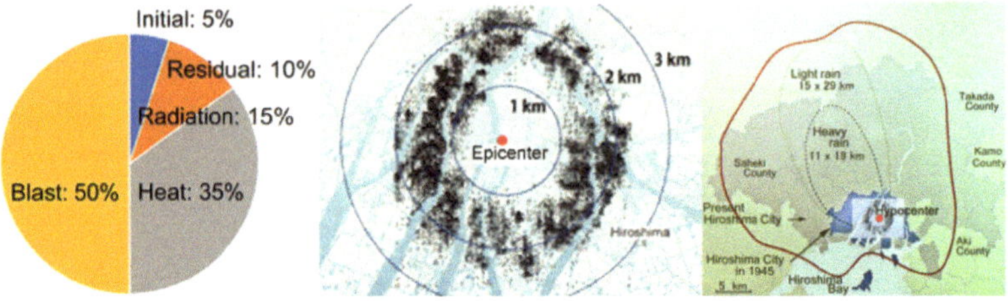

Figure 1.7 A-bomb dropped on Hiroshima and black rain. (A) Breakdown of atomic bomb energy [38]. (B) Distribution of A-bomb survivors (black dots [39]). The initial radiation range is 3 km. (C) Thick and thin dotted lines show respectively heavy and light rain areas estimated in 1953 and the thick line depicts the black rain area estimated in 2011 [40].

1.7.2 Black Rain Was Highly Radioactive

Many individuals residing beyond the 3 km radius were afflicted with acute radiation syndrome (ARS), underscoring the widespread contamination of Hiroshima City (Figs. 1.7C and 1.8A). Irrespective of indoor or outdoor exposure, those who entered the central zone within a 1 km radius of the epicenter experienced ARS, indicating severe contamination in this area (Fig. 1.8A). Furthermore, individuals who entered the city after A-bombing (NIC) also suffered from ARS, providing further evidence of significant contamination in the region (Fig. 1.8B).

1.7.3 Low Cancer Risk of A-Bomb Survivors

The Radiation Effects Research Institute (RERF) conducts a survey of A-bomb survivors as part of the Life Span Study (LSS). Mortality rates from solid cancers reported in the latest three LSS reports were compared with those for the Japanese population (Table 1.5). Cancer risk increased in the following order: NIC, A-bomb survivors, and Japanese in general. The results suggest that the residual radiation dose to which the NIC was exposed fell within the hormesis range. Most A-bomb survivors were exposed to both direct and residual radiations, but many received doses in the hormesis range and a minority received highly harmful doses. Overall, the average cancer mortality rate among survivors was lower than that of the general Japanese population who did not benefit from hormesis.

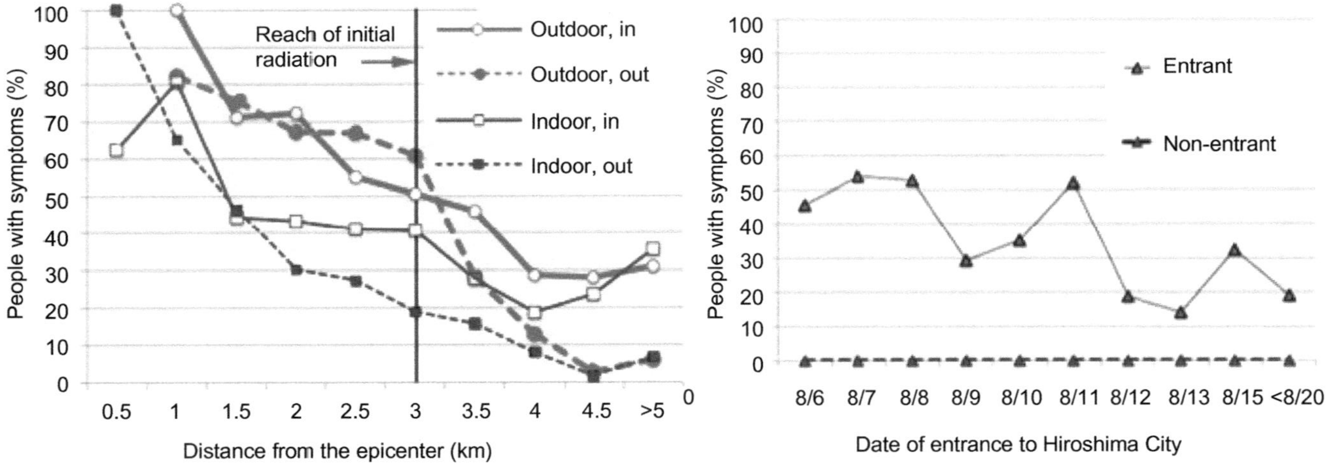

Figure 1.8 High radioactivity in black rain [41]. The initial radiation range was 3 km. (A) Number of A-bomb survivors: 398 people who entered the central area after outdoor exposure; 652 people who did not enter the area after outdoor exposure; 1,018 people who entered the area after indoor exposure; and 1,878 people who did not enter the area. (B) Number of people who entered Hiroshima City after the A-bombing (NIC): 525 people entered the central area and 104 people who did not enter the area.

Table 1.5 Solid cancer mortality in the Life Span Study (LSS) of A-bomb survivors compared with Japanese average cancer mortality [19]

Year	Survey period	No. of survivors or [NIC[a]]	No. of cancer deaths (%)	% Japanese average cancer deaths
2007	1958–1998	105,427	17,448 (16.5)	21.4 (1958–1998)
		[25,427]	[3,994 (15.7)]	
2012	1958–2000	86,611	10,929 (12.6)	22.3 (1958–2003)
		[26,529]	[NA[b]]	
2017	1958–2009	80,205	17,316 (21.6)	23.3 (1958–2009)
		[25,239]	[5,222 (20.7)]	

[a]Not-in-the-city control. [b]Not available.

1.7.4 Longer Lifespan of A-Bomb Survivors

Lifespan is a better indicator than cancer to ascertain radiation effects [42]. An LSS report has asserted that 1 Gy shortened a person's lifespan by 1.3 years [43]. However, scrutiny of the same data reveals that the dose-response of the lifespan is hormetic [19]. Early entrants who entered A-bombed cities in a month were less mortal than later entrants, suggesting more heavily exposed people lived longer (Fig. 1.9 (denoted by P)). When exposure doses were too low to categorize people by doses and they were classified by distance from the epicenter, the nearer they were to the epicenter, the less mortal they were, suggesting again that heavily exposed people lived longer (Fig. 1.9 (denoted by Q)). Of course, extensively exposed people showed shorter lifespans, but this fraction was small (6.4%). On average, A-bomb survivors lived longer. The dose response as a whole shows a J-shaped curve, a hallmark of hormesis (Fig. 1.9 (denoted by R)).

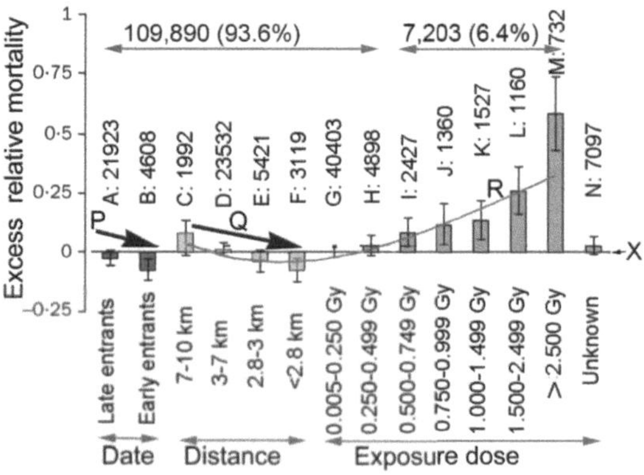

Figure 1.9 Lifespan of A-bomb survivors [19].

The Ministry of Health, Labor and Welfare is providing support to people who were directly exposed to the A-bomb in Hiroshima and Nagasaki as Category 1 Survivors. Category 2 A-bomb survivors are those who entered the area within 2 km of the hypocenter for medical treatment or to search for relatives. Those exposed to residual radioactivity fall under Category 3 survivors. Those who were fetuses of Category 1 to Category 3 survivors are defined as Category 4 survivors. The peak number of A-bomb survivors was 372,264 in 1970. The population of Japan is 124,947,000 (60,758,000 males with an average age of 81.0 and 64,189,000 females with an average age of 87.09). The weighted average is 84.15 years. On average, A-bomb survivors live about one year longer than the average Japanese (Table 1.6).

Table 1.6 Number of A-bomb survivors and average age as of March 31, 2023

Category	Number
Category 1	68,667
Category 2	22,170
Category 3	16,210
Category 4	6,602
Total	**113,649**
Average age	**85.01**

1.8 Chemical Hormesis

1.8.1 Hormesis Began with the Study of Chemical Toxicity

In 1882, a young German professor, H. Schulz discovered that disinfectants of nearly a dozen toxic agents promoted yeast growth and metabolism at low doses, but were toxic at high doses (see [44]). Southam and Ehrlich [45] coined the term "hormesis" based on the discovery that the water-soluble extractives of western red-cedar heartwood exhibited a hormesis reaction. In 1960, J.F. Townsend, T.D. Luckey [46] collected over 100 hormesis reactions from pharmaceutical journals. Subsequently, Luckey [47] summarized many hormesis reactions found in a wide range of species, including bacteria, protozoa, plants, and animals, with 1,269 references. Calabrese and Blain [48] compiled a total of approximately 900 hormetic reactions for radiation, radionuclides, inorganic compounds, and organic compounds. Research on chemical hormesis commenced 140 years ago. However, due to the vast array of chemical substances, their varied properties, diverse metabolic pathways, and other factors, the progress in chemical hormesis has lagged behind radiation hormesis.

1.8.2 Mutagen-Induced Hormetic Responses

I am one of the few members of the Japanese Environmental Mutagen and Genome Society (JEMS), which was founded in 1972. It has been commonly assumed that mutagens and carcinogens follow LNT in the same way as radiation. However, we conducted collaborative studies with the idea that there should be thresholds for the reactions caused by mutagens. Some typical examples are shown in Fig. 1.10.

In studies employing cell activity as an indicator, the dose response in TK6 cells treated with mitomycin C (MMC) showed a reverse U-shaped hormetic response (Fig. 1.10A). Similar outcomes were obtained with CHL and HeLa S3 cells.

In studies employing cell proliferation as an indicator, the dose response in L5178Y cells treated with MMC showed an inverted U-shaped hormetic response (Fig. 1.10B). Similar results were obtained when L5178Y cells were treated with ethyl methanesulfonate (EMS). TK6 cells treated with MMC also demonstrated hormesis. L5178Y cells treated with hygromycin B, aclarubicin, and colchicine also showed hormesis.

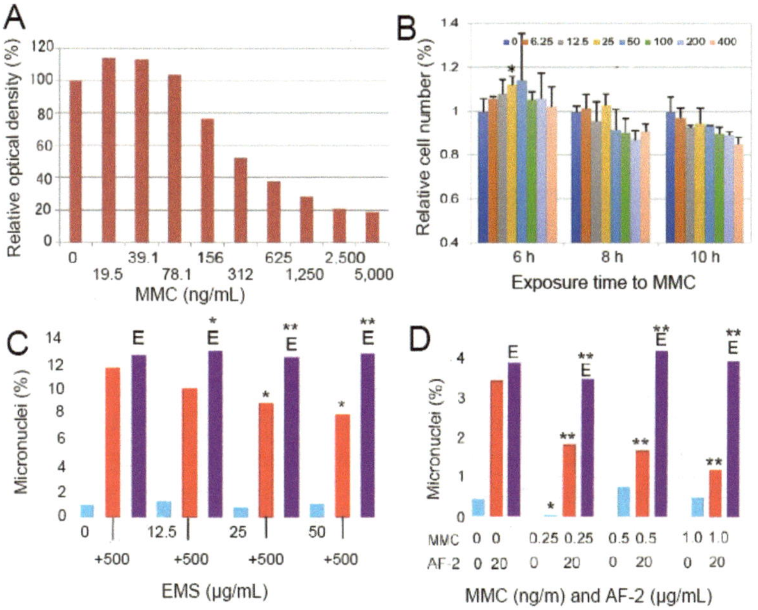

Figure 1.10 Typical examples of chemical hormesis induced by mutagens. (A) Dose-response of cell activity in TK6 cells treated with MMC [49]. (B) Dose-response of cell proliferation in L5178Y cells treated with MMC [50]. (C) Pre-treatment of L5178Y cells with a low-dose EMS, followed by treatment with a high dose of EMS [50]. (D) Micronucleus frequency when L5178Y cells were pretreated with a low dose of MMC and then treated with a high dose of AF-2 [51].

In studies focusing on micronucleus induction as an indicator, CHL cells treated with MMC showed a slightly J-shaped dose response but no statistically significant difference was obtained (data not shown). This is attributed to the inherent low incidence of micronuclei, which hovers around 1%, rendering it difficult to detect further reductions due to hormesis. Consequently, we conducted challenge tests. Specifically, L5178Y cells were initially pretreated with a low dose of EMS that does not induce micronuclei, followed by treatment 12 h later with a high dose known to induce micronuclei. This pretreatment effectively suppressed micronuclei induction (Fig. 1.10C). Parallel outcomes were observed with MMC and colchicine.

Next, cross-over tests were conducted. In this approach, cells were first pretreated with a low dose of MMC that does not induce micronuclei, followed by treatment 12 h later with a high dose of Furylfuramide (AF-2) that induces micronuclei. This sequence resulted in a suppression of micronucleus induction due to the pretreatment (Fig. 1.10D). Similar outcomes were obtained when pre-treated with AF-2 and post-treated with MMC. Similar cross-reactivity was obtained with the combination of MMC and EMS.

1.9 Discussion

Living organisms have evolved in an environment replete with radiation and chemicals since their birth. The essence of life is that it interacts with the external world and responds dynamically. These adaptive responses are inscribed in the genome. Living organisms utilize radiation to survive (Fig. 1.3). If radiation were really hazardous, we would not have survived. Hormesis is understood as part of life's fundamental adaptive responses. Radiation hormesis is ubiquitous, and several examples are shown in Fig. 1.6. Chemical hormesis brings to mind immediate examples such as vitamin deficiencies and hypervitaminosis, as well as the deleterious effects of inadequate or excessive intake of substances like salt, sugar, fat, minerals, and more. LNT, erroneously applied to radiation effects, has also been extended to mutagens. However, as depicted in Fig. 1.10, LNT is invalidated.

UV is a type of electromagnetic radiation (Fig. 1.1), which is mutagenic and can induce skin cancer when exposed in excess. Nonetheless, appropriate UV is essential for vitamin D synthesis. Radiation hormesis and chemical hormesis are not separate entities; radiation and chemicals exhibit cross-reaction [52, 53].

Although we cannot sense ionizing radiation, its main biological effect is the production of ROSs. ROSs are signaling agents detected by the Keap1-Nrf2 system. The Keap1-Nrf2 pathway is a cellular defense system against oxidative stress and xenobiotic stress stemming from

ROSs and electrophiles, respectively [54]. Upon exposure of cells to ROSs or electrophiles, Nrf2 relocates to the nucleus and triggers the transcription of more than 100 genes related to antioxidant and detoxification.

Another major pathway that deals with ROSs is the NF-κB/IκB system [55]. NF-κB proteins form a family of transcription factors that regulate the expression of hundreds of genes that play important roles not only in ROS regulation but also in processes like inflammation, immunity, cell proliferation, differentiation, development, and apoptosis. Many enzymes activated by the NF-κB/IκB system contribute to the hormetic response. Although both the Keap1-Nrf2 and NF-κB/IκB systems oversee a multitude of genes, their actions are not mutually exclusive. Many enzymes induced by the NF-κB/IκB system are involved in the hormetic reaction. For example, glutathione-S-transferase, which controls ROS levels along with enzymes such as superoxide dismutase, catalase, and glutathione peroxidase, is induced by both systems.

References

1. Sutou S. (2022) Low-dose radiation effects. *Curr. Opin. Toxicol.*, 30, 100329. https://doi.org/10.1016/j.cotox.2022.02.002
2. KamLAND Collaboration (2011) Partial radiogenic heat model for earth revealed by geoneutrino measurements. *Nature Geosci.*, 4, 647–651.
3. Jaworowski Z. (2010) Observations on the Chernobyl disaster and LNT. *Dose-Response*, 8, 148–171.
4. Muller H.J. (1927) Artificial transmutation of the gene. *Science*, 66, 84–87.
5. Sokal M.M. (1980) Science and James McKeen Cattell, 1894 to 1945. *Science*, 209, 43–52.
6. Calabrese E.J. (2018) Was Muller's 1946 Nobel Prize research for radiation-induced gene mutations peer reviewed? *Philosophy, Ethics, and Humanities in Medicine*, 2018. https://doi.org/10.1186/s13010-018-0060-5
7. Muller H.J. (1930) Radiation and genetics. *Am. Nat.*, 64, 220–251.
8. Oliver C.P. (1930) The effect of varying the duration of X-ray treatment upon the frequency of mutation. *Science*, 71, 44–46.

9. Muller H.J. http://www.nobelprize.org/nobel_prizes/medicine/laureates/1946/muller-lecture.html
10. Uphoff D.E., Stern C. (1949) The genetic effects of low intensity in irradiation. *Science*, 109, 609–610.
11. Calabrese E.J. (2023) Confirmation that Hermann Muller was dishonest in his Nobel Prize Lecture. *Arch. Toxicol.* doi: 10.1007/s00204-023-03566-5.
12. NAS (The US National Academy of Sciences) (1956) Genetic effects of atomic radiation. *Science*, 123, 1157–1164.
13. Neel J., Schull W. (1956) Studies on the potential genetic effects of the atomic bombs. *Acta Genet. Stat. Med.*, 6, 183–196.
14. Calabrese E.J. (2017) Societal threats from ideologically driven science. *Acad. Quest*, 30, 405–418.
15. Calabrese E.J., Giordano J. (2022) Ethical issues in the US 1956 National Academy of Sciences BEAR I Genetics Panel report to the public. *Health Phys.*, 123. doi: 10.1097/HP.0000000000001608.
16. NAS (The US National Academy of Sciences) (2007) Health risks from exposure to low levels of ionizing radiation: BEIR VII – Phase 2 (Free Executive Summary), 2006. http://www.philrutherford.com/Radiation_Risk/BEIR/BEIR_VII.pdf
17. Furukawa K. et al. (2015) A Bayesian semiparametric model for radiation. dose-response estimation. *Risk Analysis*, 1–13. doi: 10.1111/risa.12513
18. Sutou S. (2018) Radiation hormesis by low-dose radiation from A-bombs elongates lifespan and reduces average cancer mortality. *Sutou Genes and Environment*, 40, 26. https://doi.org/10.1186/s41021-018-0114-3
19. Sutou S. (2020) Black rain in Hiroshima: A critique to the Life Span Study of A-bomb survivors, basis of the linear no-threshold model. *Sutou Genes and Environment*, 42, 1. https://doi.org/10.1186/s41021-019-0141-8
20. ICRP. (2007) *The recommendations of the International Commission on Radiological Protection*, Publication 103, Elsevier LTD., New York.
21. Chivian D. et al. (2008) Environmental genomics reveals a single-species ecosystem deep within Earth'. *Science*, 322, 275–278.
22. Karnachuk O.V. et al. (2019) Domestication of previously uncultivated *Candidatus Desulforudis audaxviator* from a deep aquifer in Siberia sheds light on its physiology and evolution. *ISME J.*, 13, 1947–1959.

23. Flemming H.C., Wuertz S. (2019) Bacteria and archaea on Earth and their abundance in biofilms. *Nat. Rev. Microbiol.,* 17, 247–260.
24. Suzuki Y. et al. (2020) Deep microbial proliferation at the basalt interface in 33.5–104-million-year-old oceanic crust. *Commun Biol.,* 3(1), 136. doi: 10.1038/s42003-020-0860-1.
25. Sauvage J.F. et al. (2021) The contribution of water radiolysis to marine sedimentary life. *Nat Commun.,* 12(1), 1297. doi: 10.1038/s41467-021-21218-z.
26. Luckey T.D. (1986) Ionizing radiation promotes protozoan reproduction. *Radiat. Res.,* 108, 215–221.
27. Planel H. et al. (1987) Influence on cell proliferation of background radiation or exposure to very low, chronic gamma radiation. *Health Phys.,* 52, 571–578.
28. Luckey, T.D. (2007) Documented optimum and threshold for ionising radiation. *Int. J. Nuclear Law,* 1, 378–409.
29. Satta L. et al. (1995) Low environmental radiation background impairs biological defence of the yeast *Saccharomyces cerevisiae* to chemical radiomimetic agents. *Mutat. Res.,* 347, 129–133.
30. Satta L. et al. (2002) Influence of a low background radiation environment on biochemical and biological responses in V79 cells. *Radiat. Environ. Biophys.,* 41, 217–224.
31. Smith G.B. et al. (2011) Exploring biological effects of low level radiation from the other side of background. *Health Phys.,* 100, 263–265.
32. Castillo, H. et al. (2021) *Deinococcus radiodurans* UWO298 dependence on background radiation for optimal growth. *Front Genet.,* 12, 644292.
33. Castillo H. et al. (2022) Chinese hamster V79 cells' dependence on background ionizing radiation for optimal growth. *Radiat. Environ. Biophys.,* 61, 49–57.
34. Muckerheide J. (2000) It's time to tell the truth about the health benefits of low-dose radiation. *21st Century Sci. Tech.,* 13, 44–55.
35. Koana T., Tsujimura H. (2010) A U-shaped dose-response relationship between X-ray radiation and sex-linked recessive lethal mutation in male germ cells of *Drosophila. Radiat. Res.,* 174, 46–51.
36. Shimada T., Ogiu T. (1992) Effects of continuous irradiation at low-dose rates on lifespan — Philological study (II). *Radiol. Sci.,* 35, 378–383. (in Japanese)
37. Cohen B.L. (1997) Lung cancer rate vs. mean radon level in U.S. counties of various characteristics. *Health Phys.,* 72, 114–119.

38. Glaser A. (2007) Effects of nuclear weapons. http://www.princeton.edu/~aglaser/lecture2007_weaponeffects.pdf

39. Fujita, et al. (2004) DS02 survivor dose estimation at RERF. *In* Hasai et al. eds, Proceedings of the workshop *New Radiation Dosimetry System DS02 for the Atomic Bombings in Hiroshima and Nagasaki*, Research Reactor Institute, Kyoto University, pp. 142–149. http://hlweb.rri.kyoto-u.ac.jp/shibata-lab/DS02/KURRIKR114.pdf

40. Sutou, S. (2018) Low-dose radiation from A-bombs elongated lifespan and reduced cancer mortality relative to un-irradiated individuals. *Genes and Environ* 40, 26. https://doi.org/10.1186/s41021-018-0114-3

41. Sutou S. (2017) Rediscovery of an old article reporting that the area around the epicenter in Hiroshima was heavily contaminated with residual radiation, indicating that exposure doses of A-bomb survivors were largely underestimated. *J. Radiat. Res.*, 58, 745–754. https://academic.oup.com/jrr/article/58/5/745/3926493

42. Cameron J.R. (2003) Longevity is the most appropriate measure of health effects of radiation. *Radiology*, 229, 14–15.

43. Cologne J.B., Preston D.L. (2000) Longevity of atomic-bomb survivors. *Lancet*, 35, 303–307.

44. Calabrese E.J., Agathokleous E. (2020) Theodosius Dobzhansky's view on biology and evolution v.2.0: "Nothing in biology makes sense except in light of evolution and evolution's dependence on hormesis-mediated acquired resilience that optimizes biological performance and numerous diverse short and longer term protective strategies". *Environ Res.*, 186, 109559. doi: 10.1016/j.envres.2020.109559.

45. Southam C.M., Ehrlich J. (1943) Effects of extract of western red-cedar heartwood on certain wood-decaying fungi in culture. *Phytopathol.*, 33, 517–524.

46. Townsend J.F., Luckey T.D. (1960) Hormoligosis in pharmacology. *J. Amer. Med. Assoc.*, 173, 44–48.

47. Luckey TD. (2019) *Hormesis with Ionizing Radiation*, CRC Press, Boca Raton.

48. Calabrese E.J., R. Blain R. (2005) The occurrence of hormetic dose responses in the toxicological literature, the hormesis database: an overview. *Toxicol. Appl. Pharmacol.* 202, 289–301.

49. Sutou S. et al. (2018) Mammalian Mutagenicity Study Group. Collaborative study of thresholds for mutagens: Proposal of a typical protocol for detection of hormetic responses in cytotoxicity tests. *Genes Environ.*, 40, 20. doi: 10.1186/s41021-018-0108-1.

50. Sutou S. et al. (2021) Collaborative study of thresholds for mutagens. Hormetic responses in cell proliferation tests using human and murine lymphoid cells. *Dose Response.,* 19(2), 15593258211028473. doi: 10.1177/15593258211028473.

51. Sutou S. et al. (2023) Collaborative study of thresholds for mutagens: Hormetic responses in the micronucleus test and gene induction by mutagenic treatments. *Genes Environ.* (under contribution).

52. Wolff S. et al. (1988) Human lymphocytes exposed to low doses of ionizing radiations become refractory to high doses of radiation as well as to chemical mutagens that induce double-strand breaks in DNA. *Int. J. Radiat. Biol. Relat. Stud. Phys. Chem. Med.*, 53, 39–47.

53. Kakinuma S. et al. (2009) Low-dose radiation attenuates chemical mutagenesis. *Radiat. Res.* 50, 401–405.

54. Suzuki M. et al. (2016) Overview of redox regulation by Keap1–Nrf2 system in toxicology and cancer. *Curr. Opin. Toxicol.,* 1, 29–36.

55. Morgan M.J., Liu Z.G. (2011) Crosstalk of reactive oxygen species and NF-κB signaling. *Cell Res.,* 21, 103–115.

Chapter 2

The Radon Spa Controversy

Roger Rolls
Bath Medical Museum, Bath, U.K.
roger.rolls@btinternet.com

At the start of the twentieth century, many thermal springs in Europe were found to contain radioactive elements. This started a trend for popularizing radioactivity as a feature of spa treatments, particularly the administration of radon to ameliorate a variety of disorders. Only later in the century did the noxious effects of radiation start to influence doctors' attitudes toward the use of radon. Opinions were divided between those who believed radiation, no matter how small the dose, was harmful and conversely, those who believed small doses might actually have a positive health effect. The controversy still remains.

Natural thermal water has been employed for centuries in the treatment of disease. The practice is widespread and can be found in all parts of the world and often dates back to remote times, invoking legends of healing deities and special qualities not present in ordinary groundwater. Much research was done in the past to

Radioactivity in Life Sciences
Edited by Maria Letizia Terranova

ISBN 978-981-5129-67-0 (Hardcover), 978-1-003-63654-0 (eBook)
www.jennystanford.com

try to identify the nature of these healing qualities by analyzing constituents in the water that might have some therapeutic effect. Chemical elements, salts, gases, colloids, and telluric heat have all had their advocates but none has stood the test of time and advances in scientific research methodology.

Medical practitioners attached to spas have been keen to point out how the water from their springs is only efficacious if taken close to the place from which they emanate. William Oliver, an eighteenth-century physician at Bath, the UK's only hot water spa, wrote that the thermal water contained "an aetherial essence," which would be lost if it were transported elsewhere. It could not be contained in a bottle as it would pass through the cork. Cynics pointed out that if the water could be sent to the patient he or she would not need to come to Bath and the resulting fees would be lost to the physicians!

Electricity was also invoked as a possible cause of spa water's healing effect. In the mid-nineteenth century, a German chemist, Justus von Liebig was advised to visit the Austrian spa town of Gastein for treatment. Being skeptical, he analyzed the town's thermal water, which showed no evidence of being much different from his home tap water. After further medical advice, he eventually underwent the treatment and found relief. He concluded that an unknown constituent, perhaps "something electric," was responsible for this effect [1].

The idea that the Bath thermal water's therapeutic potential depended on an ethereal essence was rekindled at the start of the twentieth century when the radioactive gas radon, then known as radium emanation, was detected by Hon R.J. Strutt in 1904 in deposits taken from the King's and Hetling springs at Bath (Fig. 2.1). Radon was originally identified by Friedrich Dorn as a degradation product of radium and isolated by Ernest Rutherford and Frederick Soddy in 1902. It was recognized as a radioactive gaseous element with a very short half-life. Sir William Ramsay preferred to call the gas "niton," which translates as "shining" because the emanation given off by radium produces a glow on a zinc sulfide screen "a sort of phosphorescence that is visible in the dark" [2].

In the process of its degradation, radium releases helium nuclei as it transforms into radon. The presence of helium in spa water, first identified in 1895 by Travers and Ramsay at Cauterets, a French spa in the Hautes-Pyrenees, alerted scientists to the possible presence of radium and radon in thermal springs. Ramsay went on to analyze the thermal water of a number of European spas. Although most contained traces of radium, he found only minute quantities in the water at Bath as compared with radon, which was liberated in much larger amounts at the springs' outflow.

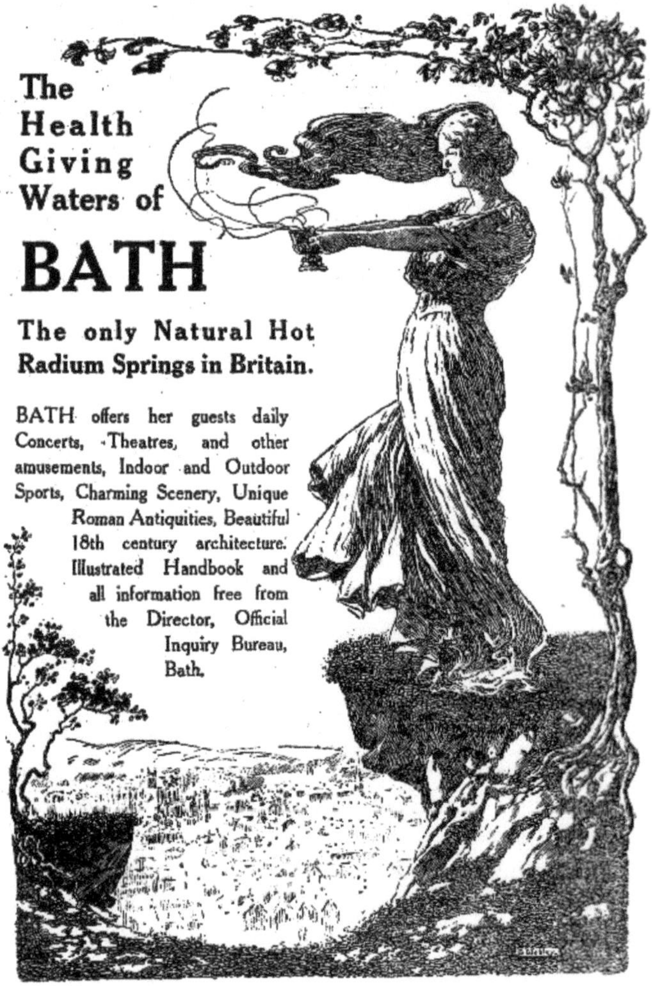

Figure 2.1 Advertisement for Radium Springs at Bath, c. 1928.

Physicians quickly became interested in the biological effects of radium and radon and were convinced that it promoted increased activity of all the processes of nutrition and metabolism. Red cells appeared to increase in number, a finding that was not observed in later experiments. Some experiments showed radon could retard the growth of microorganisms although not all researchers were able to reproduce these findings. Patients with gonorrhoeal arthritis at Bath appeared to do well after a course of spa treatment and this was thought to be due to the inhibitory action of radon on gonococci. Gout also seemed to improve with spa treatment. A German physician, Dr. F. Gudzent found in 13 out of 14 cases treated in his Berlin emanatorium, an institution for dosing patients with water infused with radon, there was a reduction in blood urate levels [3]. Conditions considered most amenable to radon treatments were musculoskeletal, skin, neoplasms, and neuralgias [4]. It has also been observed to reduce blood pressure in hypertensive patients.

Much was published on methods of administration of the naturally occurring radon. Stevenson and Ramsay at London University College Medical School fed mice with bread and cheese soaked in a solution of radon and injected kittens with the same solution and showed that the gas was eliminated via the lungs in about 3 hours. After 12 hours, all traces of the radioactive gas had disappeared. It was also believed that radon could be absorbed through the skin when subjects bathed in radioactive water. A bather would also inspire the gas, which was continually arising from the water's surface as it emerged from the springs. Ramsay suggested that as the radon gas degenerated, it would lose electrons and become positively charged. If patients receiving electric baths were connected to the negative pole of a 100-volt battery and the positive pole placed in the water, radon would theoretically accumulate on the skin, thus leading to enhanced absorption. The author added that "any experimenting on these lines would require to be made with caution and he did not know of any attempts in such a direction" [5]. It is not clear if he had tried the experiment on his kittens.

Following the discovery of natural sources of radioactivity, it became necessary to try and quantify the intensity of the radiation. Heinrich Maché introduced the first unit for radon activity levels, which was named after him (Mache-Einheit, ME) and mostly used in the German/Austrian literature, while Anglosphere countries preferred the "Curie" (Ci), introduced in 1910. Since 1975, the Becquerel (Bq) has become the preferred unit for activity [6].

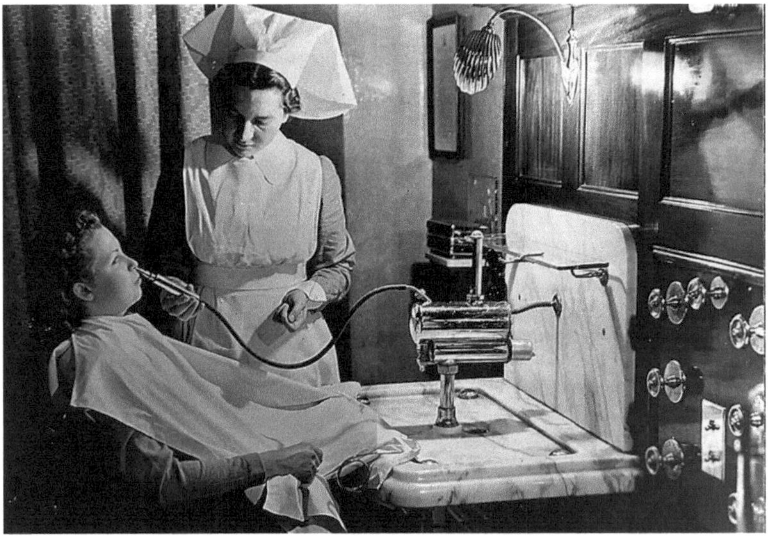

Figure 2.2 Patient in the radium inhalatorium at Bath receiving radon aerosol therapy. c. 1935, Courtesy Bath and NE Somerset Council.

Higher concentrations of radon for inhalation were achieved by using a device, which effectively atomized thermal water. At Bath Spa, radon was collected in a large metal cone suspended above the spring head. The cone was connected to a tube that ran to a room above known as an inhalatorium or emanatorium (Fig. 2.2). Radon gas and water were mixed in an apparatus producing an aerosol and fed through a flexible rubber tube to the patient's nose or mouth. Possibly the first inhalatorium to open in Europe was at Bad Kreuznach. The search was on for the most radioactive springs. Many of them are found in Japan.

Several early investigators looked for possible detrimental effects but could not find any. European spas with high radon concentration such as Gastein in Austria and Baden-Baden in Germany started to offer specific radon treatments [7].

Between 1910 and 1940, the vogue for attributing healing properties to radioactive elements led to a host of quack remedies. There were external devices like radium-impregnated bed blankets and compresses. Radium was added to drinks and food like bread, crackers, tea, and coffee (Fig. 2.3). A German patent was taken out in 1931 for radium chocolate [8] and radium "emanators" were used to make radon drinking water. All of these have been discredited as hazardous to health.

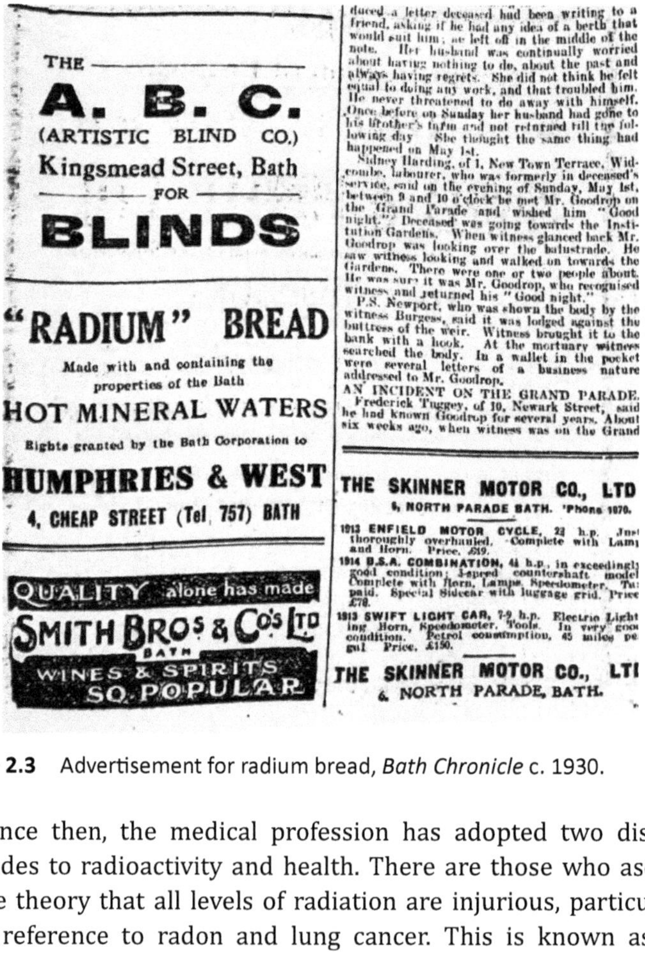

THE
A. B. C.
(ARTISTIC BLIND CO.)
Kingsmead Street, Bath
FOR
BLINDS

"RADIUM" BREAD
Made with and containing the properties of the Bath
HOT MINERAL WATERS
Rights granted by the Bath Corporation to
HUMPHRIES & WEST
4, CHEAP STREET (Tel. 757) BATH

QUALITY alone has made
SMITH BROS & CO'S LTD
BATH
WINES & SPIRITS SO POPULAR

duced a letter deceased had been writing to a friend, asking if he had any idea of a berth that would suit him; he left off in the middle of the note. Her husband was continually worried about having nothing to do, about the past and always having regrets. She did not think he felt equal to doing any work, and that troubled him. He never threatened to do away with himself. Once before on Sunday her husband had gone to his brother's farm and not returned till the following day. She thought the same thing had happened on May 1st.

Sidney Harding, of 1, New Town Terrace, Widcombe, labourer, who was formerly in deceased's service, said on the evening of Sunday, May 1st, between 9 and 10 o'clock he met Mr. Goodrop on the Grand Parade and wished him "Good night." Deceased was going towards the Institution Gardens. When witness glanced back Mr. Goodrop was looking over the balustrade. He saw witness looking and walked on towards the Gardens. There were one or two people about. He was sure it was Mr. Goodrop, who recognised witness and returned his "Good night."

P.S. Newport, who was shown the body by the witness Burgess, said it was lodged against the buttress of the weir. Witness brought it to the bank with a hook. At the mortuary witness searched the body. In a wallet in the pocket were several letters of a business nature addressed to Mr. Goodrop.

AN INCIDENT ON THE GRAND PARADE.

Frederick Tuggey, of 10, Newark Street, said he had known Goodrop for several years. About six weeks ago, when witness was on the Grand

THE SKINNER MOTOR CO., LTD
6, NORTH PARADE BATH. 'Phone 1070.

1913 ENFIELD MOTOR CYCLE, 2¾ h.p. Just thoroughly overhauled. Complete with Lamp and Horn. Price, £39.

1914 B.S.A. COMBINATION, 4¼ h.p., in exceedingly good condition; 3-speed countershaft model. Complete with Horn, Lamps, Speedometer. Tax paid. Special Sidecar with luggage grid. Price £70.

1913 SWIFT LIGHT CAR, 7-9 h.p. Electric Lighting, Horn, Speedometer, Tools. In very good condition. Petrol consumption, 45 miles per gal. Price, £150.

THE SKINNER MOTOR CO., LTD
6, NORTH PARADE, BATH.

Figure 2.3 Advertisement for radium bread, *Bath Chronicle* c. 1930.

Since then, the medical profession has adopted two distinct attitudes to radioactivity and health. There are those who ascribe to the theory that all levels of radiation are injurious, particularly with reference to radon and lung cancer. This is known as the linear no-threshold (LNT) model and is the predominant opinion in anglophone countries. The United States National Council on Radiation Protection and Measurements stated position is that ionizing radiation's effects should be considered proportional to the dose an individual receives regardless of how small that dose is. The evidence for radon exposure leading to lung cancer is uncontroversial for high levels of the gas but less clear for low levels. The lower the concentration, the lower the risk but this is assumed to be a straight-line graph. To convincingly demonstrate, there is still an increased risk of carcinogenesis with such low levels would require studies on very large cohorts of people. With regard to other malignancies, the U.K. Health Protection Agency concluded that there is insufficient evidence to suggest that radon is associated with increased risk of cancer at sites other than the lung, at low levels of radon exposure.

Opponents of the linear no-threshold model argue that the human body has defensive mechanisms, such as DNA repair and programmed cell death, which protect it against carcinogenesis from low-dose exposures to ionizing radiation. Doubt about the LNT model has been expressed by the French Academy of Sciences and the American Nuclear Society. They accept that there is scientific evidence for health risks at high dosage but exposures of less than 1 mSv are either too small to be observed or are probably non-existent. It has also been argued that the LNT model causes an irrational fear of radiation at any level and this is more injurious to health than the radiation itself.

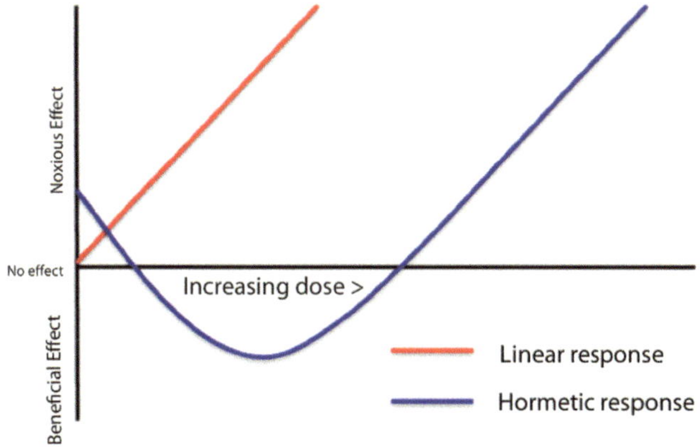

Figure 2.4 Comparison of linear no-threshold (LNT) and hormetic models of radiation exposure.

A third view, which is held by many people working in radioactive spas in mainland Europe and Russia, postulates that low doses of radiation within the region of natural background levels, or just above, are beneficial. The theory, known as radiation hormesis, proposes that low levels of radioactivity can activate cellular repair mechanisms to protect against certain diseases (Fig. 2.4).

Until the 1990s, most of the evidence for radon treatment in Central European spas was empirical but more recently controlled double-blind trials comparing natural radioactive water with carbonated tap water have been judged sufficiently reliable to stand up to scientific scrutiny. Positive effects have been reported for tendomyopathy, osteoarthritis, rheumatoid arthritis, and ankylosing spondylitis. A trial in a German spa comparing a radon-treated group of patients with rheumatoid arthritis with a control group found no observable difference in positive outcome at the end of the trial but the radon group retained their improvement at 3 and 6 months, whereas the control group quickly reverted to their pre-treatment conditions [9].

Recent basic research has helped to explain the mechanisms of radon in the human organism. It has been suggested that it is the skin that is primarily responsible for the incorporation of radon. Within its morphological structures, radiation may activate local processes that are similar to the effects of topical steroids. Animal experiments have demonstrated that the accumulation of incorporated radon, enhanced by its lipophilia, stimulates the secretion of corticoids from the adrenal cortex. Killer cell activity, which is reduced in rheumatic diseases, has been found to return to normal with radon therapy. The DNA repair capacity of the cell nucleus increases with small radiation doses, suggesting that disease-related DNA damage may be repaired more quickly and effectively. Many of these studies have been reported in foreign language journals, which may lead to ignorance by anglophone scientific communities. Certainly, in the UK, radioactivity in the thermal springs at Bath has not been mentioned in brochures since 1957 when public anxiety about radioactivity was fueled by a nuclear accident at the Windscale reprocessing plant (renamed Sellafield). A fire at the plant released radioactive elements into the atmosphere. Staff working in the spa and the Roman Baths became concerned about their radon exposure emanating from the springs and the Medical Officer of Health, Bernard Astley Weston, called upon the Radiological Protection Board to investigate. The Board calculated the radiation level around the baths and springs was 10 times lower than in Sir William Ramsay's report in 1912 and was unlikely to pose any health risk from bathing or drinking. An analysis done between 1984 and 1986 found an average level of 200

Bq/l in thermal water obtained from boreholes feeding the various baths in the spa [10]. The gas is quickly dispersed in the open air or well-ventilated rooms. Overall, the consensus remains that radon is a potential public health hazard and any reference to its presence in the thermal water of Bath might discourage people from visiting the spa baths, which are now a popular leisure facility. As for the Radium Inhalatorium, it was turned into a gift shop long ago.

Conversely, some spas in mainland Europe still advertise and promote the radioactivity of their water. "Radon spas" can be found in at least 9 EU countries. They use various arguments to support their claims. These were identified in a recent study by R. Geysmans and colleagues who found five ways in which radon spa managers "positively framed" radiation in their brochures and other promotional materials [11].

- There is experimental evidence to demonstrate health-giving effects.
- The gas is a "natural" therapy and therefore less of a perceived threat than technological therapies.
- Although there are identified risks, as there are many pharmacological therapies, the spa physician can mitigate those risks by prescribing the appropriate dose of radiation and a knowledge of contraindications.
- Radon is a special, rare, and noble gas.
- It has the power to rejuvenate, revitalize, and provide strength.

Such framing can be identified in promotional literature. For example, the spa at Bad Gastein is said to have "mild, natural radioactivity, which has exclusively beneficial effects on the body when enjoyed as part of a treatment. The noble gas radon escapes from the thermal water and thus makes its way into the body via the airways and the skin. There, it unfolds its healing properties, before being completely broken down after approximately 3 hours. This stimulates the body's defense system and the natural warmth encourages circulation" [12]. Despite these encouraging statements, the brochure adds that "the water in the thermal baths of the valley and in the spa areas of the various hotels is, incidentally, de-radonized, and can thus be enjoyed without the supervision of a doctor."

Health campaigners in the UK and USA would take issue with all of these statements. They dispute the experimental evidence, portray the gas as a major cause of indoor pollution, and focus heavily on carcinogenesis risk. Far from being "special" and rare, radon is abundant and can enter any homes, offices, schools, and buildings. And if it really is so health-promoting and safe, why bother to "de-radionize" the thermal water?

Can we draw any conclusions? It appears that the vast majority of spas with radioactive springs have negligible levels of radiation and consequently there is minimal risk, particularly when exposure is intermittent [13]. Even at Dehloran in Iran, a spa with high levels of radon, it has been calculated that visitors receive an average of 0.086 mSv per year, which is considerably below the recommended annual safe dose, although staff working regularly at this spa have a much higher annual exposure, averaging 4.89 mSv per year [14].

Thermal water generally does not pose a radiological risk for clients of spas when used for recreational purposes. There is no doubt that some patients receive benefits from spa treatment but to what extent, the presence of radon or other radioactive elements is responsible remains controversial.

References

1 Becker, K. One Century of Radon Therapy. *Int. J. Low Radiation*, Vol. 1, No. 3, 2004, p. 337.

2 Saubermann, S. Radium Emanation and Physiological Processes. *Archives of the Roentgen Ray*, Vol. 16, Issue 8, 1912, pp. 281–326.

3 Anon. Notes on the Therapeutics of Radium in the Bath Waters. Bath, 1912, p. 27.

4 Weiss, E. *On the Balneological Aspect of Radium*. Medical Press, 1912.

5 Ramsay, Sir W. Report on the Mineral Waters of Bath. Op cit Note 1.

6 For a summary of radiation units in use, see https://www.ncbi.nlm.nih.gov/books/n/nap6360/ddd0000183/

7 Aschoff, K. *Zur Einweihung des neuen Radium-Inhalatoriums*, 1912.

8 Senftner, V. Verfahren zur Herstellung radioaktiver Schokolade, German Patent 633959, Appl. 1931, issued 1936, 1931.

9 A. Franke et Al. Long-term efficacy of radon spa therapy in rheumatoid

arthritis—a randomized, sham-controlled study and follow-up. *Rheumatology*, Vol. 39, Issue 8, 2000, pp. 894–902.

10 Andrews, J.N. in Kellaway, G.A. (ed) *Hot Springs of Bath*, Bath City Council, 1991, p. 158.

11 Geysmans, R. et al. Cure or Carcinogen? A Framing Analysis of European Spa Websites. *Int. J. Public Health*, 2022. https://www.ncbi.nlm.nih.gov/pmc/articles/PMC9073685/

12 Internet advertisement, Gastein Thermal Water: https://www.salzburgerland.com/en/a-treasure-from-the-depths-of-the-mountains/

13 Dinh, C.N and Nowak J. *Natural Radioactivity in Thermal Waters: A Case Study from Poland*. https://www.mdpi.com/1996-1073/14/3/541

14 Adelikhah M et al. High Level of Natural Ionizing Radiation at a Thermal Bath in Dehloran, Iran. *Heliyon,* 6, 2020, p. e04297.

Chapter 3

Radiotherapy for Benign Conditions: Current Radiobiological and Clinical Evidence

Bruno Fionda,[a] Monica Maria Pagliara,[b] Alessandro Di Stefani,[c,d] Paolo Tropiano,[e] Francesco Bussu,[e,f] Alessio Giuseppe Morganti,[g,h] and Luca Tagliaferri[a,d]

[a]*Dipartimento di Diagnostica per Immagini e Radioterapia Oncologica, Fondazione Policlinico Universitario Agostino Gemelli IRCCS, Rome, Italy*
[b]*Dipartimento di Scienze dell'Invecchiamento, Neurologiche Ortopediche e Della Testa Collo, Fondazione Policlinico Universitario Agostino Gemelli IRCCS, Rome, Italy*
[c]*Dipartimento di Scienze Mediche e Chirurgiche, Fondazione Policlinico Universitario Agostino Gemelli IRCCS, Rome, Italy*
[d]*Università Cattolica del Sacro Cuore, Rome, Italy*
[e]*Division of Otolaryngology, Azienda Ospedaliero-Universitaria, Sassari, Italy*
[f]*Department of Medicine, Surgery and Pharmacology, University of Sassari, Sassari, Italy*
[g]*Radiation Oncology, IRCCS Azienda Ospedaliero-Universitaria di Bologna, Bologna, Italy*
[h]*Department of Experimental, Diagnostic and Specialty Medicine-DIMES, Alma Mater Studiorum University of Bologna, Bologna, Italy*
bruno.fionda@policlinicogemelli.it

Radioactivity in Life Sciences
Edited by Maria Letizia Terranova

ISBN 978-981-5129-67-0 (Hardcover), 978-1-003-63654-0 (eBook)
www.jennystanford.com

3.1 Introduction to Radiotherapy for Benign Conditions

The use of radiotherapy (RT) for benign conditions (also called benign disorders or benign tumors) has a solid scientific background and roughly 40000 patients have been included in clinical reports to have received RT as part of their treatment strategy for a benign condition [1].

A comprehensive review of all the known indications from a historical perspective allowed us to identify over 100 clinical benign disorders that could benefit from the use of RT [2].

Since the number of clinical situations is so elevated, several attempts have been to propose different classification systems in order to frame all of them. The Royal College of Radiologists in the United Kingdom organized the different conditions according to the primary anatomical sites involving eyes, bones and joints, head and neck, skin, brain, heart, and peripheral vessels [3].

Another interesting approach is the one proposed by the German Cooperative Group on Radiotherapy for Benign Diseases, which proposed to organize the indications according to the underlying physiopathological mechanisms into five main categories: degenerative diseases, hyperproliferative diseases, functional diseases, stereotactic indications, and rare indications [4].

A worldwide survey performed within the clinical community was published in 1998 and allowed us to draw some interesting conclusions; in fact, 508 different institutions from all over the world shared their protocols with a particular focus on indications and RT schedules. It clearly emerged from the results of this survey that there was a significant variability both in terms of indications of clinical conditions treated and RT schedules used across the responding institutions. One of the most relevant points of discussion was that such significant differences in clinical practice were related to the different geographical origins of the institutions. Therefore, this finding urged the need for further research to reach a more homogenous approach to the topic [5].

3.2 The Radiobiological Rationale

The understanding of how RT might contribute to treating benign conditions is quite recent. Even though RT has always been used to treat inflammatory conditions, early clinicians did not have enough data to realize the radiobiological rationale [6].

The main point to consider is that macrophages, one of the key players in the immune system, are sensitive to ionizing radiation such as X-rays and γ-rays. Their sensitivity is important because it affects a delicate balance in the macrophage polarization between different phenotypes: namely M1-like and M2-like. In particular, the M2 polarization is associated with a reduction in the inflammatory response, and therefore, with the benefit of RT in benign conditions. Such polarization is triggered by several chemical stimuli (such as a decrease of reactive oxygen species and nitric oxide levels) and cytokines (the suppression of TNF-α and the increase of TNF-β) [7].

Another point of paramount relevance is the role of fibroblasts, which are cells involved in extracellular matrix maintenance within healthy human tissues. Ionizing radiations typically induce a level of ROS production that could exceed the threshold to inhibit the proliferation of fibroblasts, thus further contributing to reducing inflammation levels [8].

Another relevant aspect to take into account from the radiobiological point of view is the risk of radiation-induced cancers following exposure to radiotherapy for benign conditions. The evidence for the magnitude of such risk derives from different scientific reports and suffers from the fact that there are only a few long-term follow-up studies covering this topic. On the whole, the available evidence suggests that the risks of radiation-induced cancer following RT for benign diseases are low, especially in older patients; obviously when dealing with young patients a careful balance between risk and benefit should be considered before proposing any radiation treatment [9].

3.3 Current Indications and Evidence Supporting the Clinical Practice

A recent review of literature aimed at providing the level of evidence for all main indications, according to the Oxford Levels of Evidence. This scale includes several levels of clinical evidence as follows [10]:

Table 3.1 Classification of commonly accepted radiotherapy indication in the clinical practice for benign disorders

		Functional category			
		Degenerative	**Hyperproliferative**	**Functional**	**Stereotactic**
Anatomical site	**Eye**		Pterygium (1a)*	Graves' disease (1a)* Orbital pseudotumor (4)*	
	Head and neck		Pleomorphic adenoma (3a)*	Sialorrhoea (4)*	Paraganglioma (4)*
	Skin		Keloid (1a)*	Lymphatic fistula (4)*	
	Brain				Arteriovenous malformation (1b)* Meningioma (1a)* Acoustic neuroma (2a)* Pituitary adenoma (4)* Trigeminal neuralgia (4)*
	Bones and joints	Arthritis (1a)* Tendinitis (1b)*	Dupuytren's disease (1b)* Ledderhose's disease (4)*	Heterotopic ossification (1a)*	
	Heart and peripheral vascular system			Coronary stent restenosis (1a)* Vascular stent restenosis (1a)*	Refractory cardiac arrhythmias (4) *
Dose range (Gy)		2–8	3–30	6–40	12–60

**Level of evidence according to the Oxford Levels of Evidence*

- Level 1a includes systematic reviews of randomized controlled trials
- Level 1b includes individual randomized controlled trials
- Level 2a includes systematic reviews of cohort studies
- Level 2b includes individual cohort study
- Level 3a includes systematic reviews of case-control studies
- Level 3b includes individual case-control studies
- Level 4 includes case-series
- Level 5 includes expert opinions

Table 3.1 summaries all the current clinical indications for RT in benign disorders, and it is noteworthy that most indications are supported by a very high level of evidence [11].

Since the number of indications for RT in benign disorders includes several anatomical districts and different schedules (doses and fractionations), we will provide an insight into some clinical examples that are representatives of the other conditions; in detail, we will focus on specific conditions affecting the eyes (and the orbital region) as well as the head and neck (H&N) region.

3.4 Clinical Examples

3.4.1 The Role of Radiotherapy in Pterygium

Pterygium represents an ocular surface pathological condition in which patients suffer from a wing-shaped growth of limbal and conjunctival tissue, within the palpebral fissure; the tissue growth progressively involves the cornea. Regarding the risk factors that have been identified in the development of pterygium, we may take into account several factors such as demographic, environmental, and lifestyle factors.

However, the most relevant risk factor that is involved both in the pathogenies and the progression of pterygium is the exposure of patients to UV light. The prevalence greatly varies according to the different geographic locations ranging from low incidence in some areas (1%) to higher prevalence (over 30% in some circumstances).

From a clinical point of view, pterygium is typically asymptomatic; however, patients may suffer from disruption of tear film, due to eye irritation secondary to dryness triggered by inflammation of the tissue. In more advanced conditions, tissue growth could be associated with visus alteration (patients could turn out to be astigmatic). The cornea might be flattened following the direction of the growing pterygium, and this finding is particularly frequent in the case of lesions with a diameter superior to 2 mm. In the late stages, the pterygium may significantly affect the visus, especially in those cases where, by invading the cornea, the lesion results in the cornea's optical center obscuration.

Talking about therapeutic options for pterygium, the available evidence suggests that a simple surgical excision could result in an unacceptable recurrence rate (ranging from 24% to 89%), and therefore, adjuvant treatments should be considered after the surgical removal of the primary lesion.

There are several adjuvant options, which have been explored with good results in the clinical practice including conjunctival-limbar autograft or topical medications (including cyclosporine, mitomycin C, 5-fluorouracil, or bevacizumab). These choices are associated with a recurrence rate of roughly 5–10%. Also, adjuvant irradiation, delivered immediately after surgery, may effectively reduce the risk of pterygium recurrence and is a valid alternative to other medical adjuvant options.

RT is a well-established option and a comprehensive literature review was able to identify over 6,000 patients treated by RT over the years. Pterygium is one of the clinical situations in which we may find even prospective randomized trials, even though most of the available clinical evidence comes from retrospective reports.

The typical radiotherapy technique used for pterygium implies the use of a β-emitter epibulbar applicator (such as strontium-90), which is adapted as closely as possible to the treatment.

In the adjuvant treatment of pterygium, it is important to deliver the first fraction as soon as possible, if possible, even within a few hours after the excision.

With regard to the schedules currently accepted, there is a great variety of regimens ranging from 20 Gy in one single fraction to 60 Gy in 6 fractions; however, the largest and most recent reports available in literature used 30–35 Gy in 3, 5, or 7 fractions [12].

3.4.2 The Role of Radiotherapy in Orbital Pseudotumor

Orbital pseudotumor (or pseudotumor orbital) is a benign disorder that is also known among clinicians as an idiopathic orbital inflammatory syndrome (IOIS), which groups together a long series of several benign space-occupying lesions affecting the orbit.

From the epidemiological point of view, IOIS may affect patients of all ages and overall accounts for almost 6% of all orbital diseases; in statistical terms, it is the third most common cause of orbital disease, after thyroid-associated conditions and lymphoproliferative diseases.

When analyzing the typical clinical presentation IOIS normally is associated with a subacute onset of painful proptosis and periorbital tissue inflammation; with regard to laterality, symptoms are most cases unilateral but a bilateral presentation is far from rare in clinical practice.

Over the decades, different classification systems based on histopathological examination have been proposed but still nowadays, the term IOSI remains a nosologic umbrella including different clinical and pathological situations that could not otherwise be classified.

The management of IOIS plays a role of paramount relevance because, even though benign, this condition may in selected circumstances be associated with severe morbidity in terms of inflammatory symptoms with consequent visus reduction.

Treatment approaches traditionally imply the use of steroids; however, also nonsteroidal anti-inflammatory drugs, chemotherapy, and immunotherapy have been widely investigated in recent studies. In highly selected patients who are affected by a refractory disease, radiotherapy (RT) could play a role in management because irradiation has been shown to be effective in suppressing the inflammatory process. RT could be considered also in those cases in which the clinical comorbidities or the presence of side effects could be limiting factors for additional systemic therapies.

A recent systematic review identified data from 241 patients published in the literature, who received RT for IOIS.

The response rate in this report ranged from 74% to 100% with a median recurrence rate of only 10%; with regard to the time required for the treatment to obtain the expected positive effects, they were clinically present within 1–2 months from the end of RT in most of the cases.

The median total dose delivered to the orbital target was 20 Gy and the most commonly reported fractionation was 2 Gy per day in most of the reports; however, lower (0.5 Gy twice weekly) and higher (5 Gy per day) doses/fractions have also been described [13].

3.4.3 The Role of Radiotherapy in Schwannomas

Schwannomas are uncommon and benign lesions that encapsulate nerve sheath with a slow-growing are called this way because they arise from Schwann cells. Alternative names currently used in the scientific literature are neuro schwannoma, neurilemmoma, and Verocay's neuroma.

Schwannomas may occur along any cranial, peripheral, or autonomic nerve in the entire body, with the exception of the olfactory and optic nerves because these last two nerves do not have Schwann cells. Roughly 25–45% of schwannomas are usually diagnosed within the extracranial region of the head and neck and typically arise in the lateral part of the neck. Neck schwannomas could be further subdivided into medial or lateral. Schwannomas originating in the medial part of the neck include those arising from the cervical sympathetic chain or the last four cranial nerves namely the glossopharyngeal, the vagus, the accessory, and the hypoglossal. Schwannomas arising in the lateral part of the neck are those originating from the trunk of the cervical or brachial plexus. A very common intracranial site of origin for schwannomas is the acoustic nerve.

From the clinical point of view, schwannomas are usually asymptomatic. Specific symptoms however may be associated according to the nerve of origin of the tumor. For example, in the case of an extracranial tumor such in the case of vagal schwannomas, one of the most frequently reported symptoms is hoarseness of the voice, which is secondary to the paralysis of the vocal cords. Sometimes patients with vagal schwannomas could even suffer from paroxysmal cough if the tumor is touched and this last finding is highly suggestive of the origin of the vagal nerve. In more advanced cases of vagal schwannomas, when the size of the lesion is considerable, further symptoms could develop, including dysphagia, hoarseness, pharyngeal, or airway obstruction with related dyspnea.

When considering an intracranial tumor, like in the case of acoustic nerve schwannomas, the typical presentation includes unilateral hearing loss, tinnitus, and vertigo in the early stages; in more advanced stages, headache, double vision, ataxia, and dysphagia could be reported.

Regarding the therapeutic options, complete surgical removal is the treatment of choice in these tumors; however, the clinical management of schwannomas requires a multidisciplinary evaluation. Often, the diagnostic pathway is challenging, due to the indolent growth and the lack of pathognomonic symptoms and the therapeutic management should take into account the general clinical conditions and comorbidities.

Radiotherapy could be considered a therapeutic option in cases of patients unfit for surgery and with a symptomatic clinical presentation in vagal schwannomas [14].

Considering lesions arising in the intracranial setting such as vestibular schwannoma, RT plays a more relevant role in the treatment strategy. Indeed, in small vestibular schwannoma lesions, stereotaxic RT may allow for similar local control and potentially better functional outcomes than surgery, and in the case of large and irregularly shaped lesions, standard RT may be considered for patients non-surgical [15].

3.4.4 The Role of Radiotherapy in Kimura's Disease

Kimura's disease (KD) is a benign disorder characterized by the presence of a subcutaneous mass typically arising in the H&N region. From an epidemiological point of view, it mostly arises in young people of Asian origin, with the highest incidence between the second and third decades of life. However, KD may also occur in other ethnic groups and it is not uncommon to affect children.

Regarding the etiology of KD, this disorder is always associated with chronic inflammatory lesions but the precise causes remain unsolved.

Several attempts have been made in order to find possible associations and some researchers have proposed a possible interference among allergic reactions, viral, or parasitic (even with arthropod bites) with the immune system. In some circumstances, KD might be associated with multiple organ involvement, and renal function impairment is a common finding in these patients. Other systemic conditions have been studied and reported to be possibly associated with KD including hepatitis, cardiovascular disease, and asthma.

When considering treatment strategies that are described in the medical literature, we may list both systemic and locoregional options; the most commonly used drugs are steroids and mitomycin C. However, the most frequently used locoregional treatment is by far surgical management, which could be followed in selected cases by postoperative RT; in some cases, RT has been used also as an alternative to surgery as the primary approach.

A recent systematic review reported data published in the literature about 124 patients.

Most patients treated by RT were aged between 10 and 30 years and were mostly male. The mean follow-up time ranged from 1.5 to 13 years.

In some series mainly the older ones, RT was prescribed as exclusive treatment in some cases. However, in the most recent and numerous reports, RT has been used as postoperative therapy. The median largest size of treated lesions was 9.5 cm.

The response rate in unresected patients ranged from 92.9% to 100% and the median recurrence rate across all the patients was 11%.

The RT schedules used in the different series were not uniform. The doses delivered ranged from 13 Gy to 56 Gy. However, in the majority of reports presenting these data, the delivered dose was between 20 Gy and 45 Gy with standard fractionation [16].

3.4.5 The Role of Radiotherapy in Pleomorphic Adenoma

Pleomorphic adenoma (PA) is, together with cystoadenolymphoma (Warthin tumor), the most common benign tumor of the salivary glands [17, 18]. The main treatment option is for sure surgery, with a very high control rate in primary cases; if the surgical technique is careful and appropriate, around 99% in the best series [19–21].

However, even if it is histologically benign, PA management is much trickier than that of Warthin tumors, mainly for the following reasons:

It is generally hard consistency and the tendency to grow around the facial nerve branches, which lie in grooves along the tumor tends to make the dissection from the nerve itself much more difficult.

This latter fact, combined with less favorable biology and the absence of a real capsule (pseudo capsule) makes rupture spillage and recurrence much more common. Such recurrences are typically multifocal.

AP has a relevant malignant transformation rate (5.9% among primary cases and 20.0% among recurrent cases) usually in very aggressive carcinomas ex-pleomorphic adenomas, with a clear propensity to nerve invasion and most of all distant metastasis [21, 22].

For this reason, the primary surgery for pleomorphic adenoma must be a safe complete resection, that is, in case of an origin from the parotid, a wide resection along the plane of the facial nerve and wherever possible a large cuff of normal salivary tissue around the lesion (parotidectomy). This is a completely different concept from extracapsular dissection, which bears unacceptable risks of recurrence [23].

In fact, recurrent PA is a challenging clinical scenario without current high-level evidence (retrospective studies, level 3a) to guide clinical decisions.

Several works strongly suggest that radiotherapy can play a role. Both photons and neutrons (hadrontherapy) have been employed [24, 25].

Limitations of current studies are that the clinical situations for indications of radiotherapy have not been standardized.

According to some authors [18, 26] radiotherapy may be considered in cases of incomplete surgical resection before recurrence, but this event should be avoided through appropriate indications and surgical technique.

In the case of recurrent PA, if the tumor cannot be completely removed due to its location, multiple nodules (often tens), and/or the risk of damaging critical structures (mainly facial nerve) radiotherapy seems to be an option, in general, in combination with facial nerve-sparing surgery.

In fact, several studies describe a better local control of recurrent PA, with surgery and postoperative radiotherapy than with surgery alone [18, 24, 25, 27–31].

Few other studies [32] argue on the contrary that RT does not significantly influence tumor control.

To our knowledge, no comparison is available between photons and neutrons in pleomorphic adenomas. However, neutrons are often advocated for their effectiveness against salivary gland malignancies and have been described to have a promisingly high local control rate (76%) in gross residual disease even if the long-term grade III/IV toxicity rate is high (21%) [24].

In general, although evidence suggests that the integration of radiation therapy can play a relevant role in managing RPA, it should be kept in mind that radiotherapy carries potential risks and side effects, and patients who receive radiotherapy will require any long-term follow-up and monitoring, besides treatment response and potential recurrence, also late-term side effects of radiation therapy.

In conclusion, radiotherapy can play a role in the management of recurrent pleomorphic adenoma, particularly in cases of incomplete surgical resection, multiple recurrences, or palliative treatment. However, its use should be carefully evaluated and individualized for each patient based on their specific clinical situation and the expertise of the Institution.

References

1. Fionda B, Lancellotta V, Casà C, Boldrini L, Marazzi F, Cellini F, Kovács G, Gambacorta MA, Tagliaferri L. Radiotherapy for benign disorders: current use in clinical practice. *Eur Rev Med Pharmacol Sci.*, 2021, 25(9), 3440–3443. doi: 10.26355/eurrev_202105_25824
2. Order SE, Donaldson SS. *Radiation Therapy of Benign Diseases: A Clinical Guide*, 2003. ISBN 978-3-540-00575-9
3. The Royal College of Radiologists. A review of the use of radiotherapy in the UK for the treatment of benign clinical conditions and benign tumors. *Clin Oncol.*, 2015. ISBN 978-1-905034-66-6
4. Kriz J, Seegenschmiedt HM, Bartels A, Micke O, Muecke R, Schaefer U, Haverkamp U, Eich HT. Updated strategies in the treatment of benign diseases: patterns of care study of the German cooperative group on benign diseases. *Adv Radiat Oncol.*, 2018, 3(3), 240–244. doi: 10.1016/j.adro.2018.02.008

5. Leer JW, van Houtte P, Davelaar J. Indications and treatment schedules for irradiation of benign diseases: a survey. *Radiother Oncol.*, 1998, 48(3), 249–257. doi: 10.1016/s0167-8140(98)00051-6
6. Frey B, Hehlgans S, Rödel F, Gaipl US. Modulation of inflammation by low and high doses of ionizing radiation: implications for benign and malign diseases. *Cancer Lett.*, 2015, 368(2), 230–237. doi: 10.1016/j.canlet.2015.04.010
7. Calabrese EJ, Dhawan G, Kapoor R, Kozumbo WJ. Radiotherapy treatment of human inflammatory diseases and conditions: optimal dose. *Hum Exp Toxicol.*, 2019, 38(8), 888–898. doi: 10.1177/0960327119846925
8. Rödel F, Fournier C, Wiedemann J, Merz F, Gaipl US, Frey B, Keilholz L, Seegenschmiedt MH, Rödel C, Hehlgans S. Basics of radiation biology when treating hyperproliferative benign diseases. *Front Immunol.*, 2017, 8, 519. doi: 10.3389/fimmu.2017.00519
9. McKeown SR, Hatfield P, Prestwich RJ, Shaffer RE, Taylor RE. Radiotherapy for benign disease: assessing the risk of radiation-induced cancer following exposure to intermediate dose radiation. *Br J Radiol.*, 2015, 88(1056), 20150405. doi: 10.1259/bjr.20150405
10. https://www.cebm.ox.ac.uk/resources/levels-of-evidence/oxford-centre-for-evidence-based-medicine-levels-of-evidence-march-2009
11. Fionda B, Rembielak A. Is there still a role for radiation therapy in the management of benign conditions? *Clin Oncol (R Coll Radiol)*, 2022, S0936-6555(22)00460-5. doi: 10.1016/j.clon.2022.09.051
12. Fionda B, Pagliara MM, Jaberi R. *The GEC ESTRO Handbook of Brachytherapy*, 2nd edition, 2023. Chapter 33: Pterygum.
13. Fionda B, Pagliara MM, Lancellotta V, Sammarco MG, Casà C, Savino G, Deodato F, Morganti AG, Gambacorta MA, Tagliaferri L, Blasi MA. The role of radiotherapy in orbital pseudotumor: a systematic review of literature. *Ocul Immunol Inflamm.*, 2022, 30(5), 1162–1167. doi: 10.1080/09273948.2020.1871493
14. Loperfido A, Celebrini A, Fionda B, Bellocchi G, Cristalli G. Diagnostic and therapeutic strategy for vagal schwannoma: case series and literature review. *Medicina (Kaunas)*, 2023, 59(6), 1013. doi: 10.3390/medicina59061013
15. Apicella G, Paolini M, Deantonio L, Masini L, Krengli M. Radiotherapy for vestibular schwannoma: a review of recent literature results. *Rep Pract Oncol Radiother.*, 2016, 21(4), 399–406. doi: 10.1016/j.rpor.2016.02.002

16. Fionda B, Loperfido A, Bussu F, Lancellotta V, Casà C, Vavassori A, Vicenzi L, Re A, Deodato F, Morganti AG, Gambacorta MA, Tagliaferri L. The role of radiotherapy in Kimura's disease: a multicenter systematic review of literature. *Eur Rev Med Pharmacol Sci.*, 2021, 25(12), 4205–4210. doi: 10.26355/eurrev_202106_26124
17. Fois P, Mureddu L, Manca A, Varrucciu S, Crescio C, Gallus R, Rizzo D, Cossu A, Bussu F. Preoperative diagnosis of Warthin tumors combining cytological, clinical and ultrasonographic information within a multidisciplinary approach in a lump clinic. *J Pers Med.*, 2023, 13(7), 1075. doi: 10.3390/jpm13071075
18. Wallace AS, Morris CG, Kirwan JM, Werning JW, Mendenhall WM. Radiotherapy for pleomorphic adenoma, *Am J Otolaryngol.*, 2013, 34(1), 36–40. doi: 10.1016/j.amjoto.2012.08.002
19. Laccourreye H, Laccourreye O, Cauchois R, et al. Total conservative parotidectomy for primary benign pleomorphic adenoma of the parotid gland: a 25-year experience with 229 patients. *Laryngoscope,* 1994, 104, 1487–1494.
20. Myssiorek D, Ruah CB, Hybels RL. Recurrent pleomorphic adenomas of the parotid gland. *Head Neck,* 1990, 12, 332–336.
21. Choi SY, Choi J, Hwang I, Cho J, Ko YH, Jeong HS. Comparative longitudinal analysis of malignant transformation in pleomorphic adenoma and recurrent pleomorphic adenoma. *J Clin Med.*, 2022, 11(7), 1808. doi: 10.3390/jcm11071808
22. Bussu F, Parrilla C, Rizzo D, Almadori G, Paludetti G, Galli J. Clinical approach and treatment of benign and malignant parotid masses, personal experience. *Acta Otorhinolaryngol Ital.*, 2011, 31(3), 135–143.
23. Kanatas A, Ho MWS, Mücke T. Current thinking about the management of recurrent pleomorphic adenoma of the parotid: a structured review. *Br J Oral Maxillofac Surg.*, 2018, 56(4), 243–248. doi: 10.1016/j.bjoms.2018.01.021
24. Douglas JG, Einck J, Austin-Seymour M, Koh WJ, Laramore GE. Neutron radiotherapy for recurrent pleomorphic adenomas of major salivary glands. *Head Neck,* 2001, 23(12), 1037–1042. doi: 10.1002/hed.10027
25. Becelli R, Morello R, Renzi G, Matarazzo G, Dominici C. Recurrent pleomorphic adenoma of the parotid gland: role of neutron radiation therapy. *J Craniofac Surg.*, 2012, 23(5), e449–e450. doi: 10.1097/SCS.0b013e318262d291
26. Witt RL, Eisele DW, Morton RP, Nicolai P, Poorten VV, Zbären P. Etiology and management of recurrent parotid pleomorphic adenoma. *Laryngoscope,* 2015, 125(4), 888–893. doi: 10.1002/lary.24964

27. Liu FF, Rotstein L, Davison AJ, et al. Benign parotid adenomas: a review of the Princess Margaret Hospital experience. *Head Neck*, 1995, 17, 177–183.
28. Dawson AK. Radiation therapy in recurrent pleomorphic adenoma of the parotid. *Int J Radiat Oncol Biol Phys.*, 1989, 16, 819–821.
29. Chen AM, Garcia J, Bucci MK, et al. Recurrent pleomorphic adenoma of the parotid gland: long-term outcome of patients treated with radiation therapy. *Int J Radiat Oncol Biol Phys.*, 2006, 66, 1031–1035.
30. Samson MJ, Meson R, Wang CC, Montgomery WW. Preservation of the facial nerve in the management of recurrent pleomorphic adenoma. *Laryngoscope*, 1991, 101(10), 1060–1062. doi: 10.1288/00005537-199110000-00006
31. Renehan A, Gleave EN, McGurk M. An analysis of the treatment of 114 patients with recurrent pleomorphic adenomas of the parotid gland. *Am J Surg.*, 1996, 172, 710–714.
32. Yugueros P, Goellner JR, Petty PM, Woods JE. Treating recurrence of parotid benign pleomorphic adenomas. *Ann Plast Surg.*, 1998, 40(6), 573–576. doi: 10.1097/00000637-199806000-00001

Chapter 4

Ultra-High-Dose Rate FLASH Radiotherapy

Gaia Franciosini, Lucia Giuliano, Luigi Palumbo, and Vincenzo Patera
Dipartimento di Scienze di Base applicate per l'ingegneria, Università La Sapienza, Roma, Italy
lucia.giuliano@uniroma1.it

4.1 Introduction

The treatment of cancer can take advantage of different strategies, applied singularly or in combination: surgery, chemotherapy, and external beam radiotherapy (EBRT). The latter can be exploited using different radiation sources: generally, X-rays are used. Also, electrons, protons, and carbon ions are present in clinical practice. The main challenge of EBRT is the accurate administration of the tumor lesion of the needed dose (defined in Gy as the ratio of energy released to a tissue volume concerning its mass) while minimizing the amount of ionizing radiation given to the surrounding healthy

Radioactivity in Life Sciences
Edited by Maria Letizia Terranova

ISBN 978-981-5129-67-0 (Hardcover), 978-1-003-63654-0 (eBook)
www.jennystanford.com

tissue. The quest for better tumor control probability (TCP), reducing the Normal Tissues Complications (NTC), and increasing the expectancy and quality of life of the patients, led radiotherapy (RT) to continuous and fast development over the past 50 years.

EBRT treatments usually span over several weeks, with irradiation sessions occurring several times per week. The overall duration of the therapy may also change due to factors such as the specific tumor type and the patient's response to therapy. In conventional EBRT, each irradiation session can last a few minutes, and the dose administered can fall within the range of 1–6 Gy.

The described complex fractionation scheme has its roots in two opposite needs: eradicate the cancer cells while giving enough time to the healthy tissue to recover from radiation damage during the interval between two treatment fractions. Despite a certain level of tolerance to the radiation toxicity of healthy tissues, achieving a successful treatment with zero complications probability is an unattainable goal. Treatment prescription is a careful trade-off between potential risks and attainable benefits. This delicate equilibrium is defined as the therapeutic window. Figure 4.1 shows the probability of effective tumor control (TC, green solid line), together with the probability of adverse events in healthy tissue, due to radiation toxicity (NTC, red solid line). The difference between these two probabilities is shown by the blue solid line and is named the "therapeutic window." In other words, the therapeutic window encompasses the range of doses that optimize anti-tumor efficacy while keeping radio-induced toxicity at an acceptable level.

The mechanistic understanding of radiation interactions with matter, the planning of the treatments that rely on the available diagnostic/imaging information, the delivery of the radiation beam to the patient, and the treatment monitoring to ensure that the entire protocol proceeds as planned, are areas of continuous research to maximize the therapy performance and reduce the cost/benefit ratio.

In this context, in the last decade, experimental evidence is growing about the possibility of achieving NCTP reduction delivering the dose at much higher rates (hundreds of times or more) than the current clinical practice. This so-called 'FLASH effect' has the potential to reshape the future of RT, in particular for charged beam treatments.

FLASH irradiation is characterized by extremely short delivery times, typically on the order of 10 milliseconds. Unlike conventional RT, FLASH RT aims ideally to deliver the entire dose in a single fraction. Must be underlined that the FLASH approach appears to spare healthy tissues from ionizing radiation damage while maintaining the same efficacy in tumor eradication with respect to conventional RT. As a consequence, in Fig. 4.1, it can be observed a remarkable rightward shift in the NTCP curve for FLASH irradiation (red dashed line), while the TCP curve (green dashed line) remains unchanged compared to conventional irradiation.

This experimental evidence has sparked excitement within the RT research community for the possibility provided by the FLASH effect to have more effective treatments delivered in shorter time intervals. Such a paradigm shift holds the promise of a significant improvement in the post-treatment quality of life for many oncological patients.

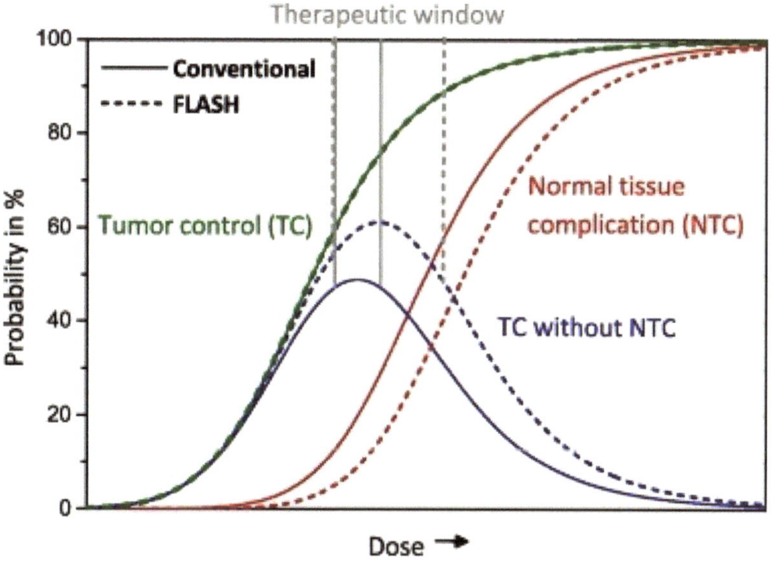

Figure 4.1 Illustration of dependence of tumor control probability (green) and normal tissue complications probability (red) on dose for conventional (solid) and FLASH (dashed) radiotherapy. In blue, there is the therapeutic window (Schuller et al. [1]).

However, the evidence collected so far about the FLASH effect asks for substantial research activity to be consolidated before translating the FLASH irradiation into the clinic. The quoted sparing effect has been demonstrated using both in vivo and in vitro experiments [2–5], despite the very few facilities around the world that are currently able to deliver beams with the required FLASH parameters [6–8]. There is a huge need for more facilities to allow a wider scientific community to perform the needed biological studies on cells, tissues, and organs (in small animals), as well as preclinical tests exploiting different beam types and energies.

The beam intensity needed to achieve the FLASH rates is so high that standard monitoring and dosimetry techniques used in the clinical routine may fail in precisely measuring the absorbed dose and its rate. An example of the new effect introduced by such a high-dose rate is the ion recombination effects that heavily affect ionization chambers limiting their precision in the FLASH regime [9]. On top of that, most of the experiments have been carried out so far in a simplified setup (e.g., a single field of radiation at a fixed energy and position), and further effects could be presented in realistic operations.

To consistently deal with all challenges of the FLASH effect implementation in clinical practice, the biological mechanism understanding and modeling of the effect plays a crucial role, together with the necessary research and development in the acceleration and beam delivery technology, needed to provide the required dose rates with clinically acceptable precision. A final word on the FLASH effect will be said only if novel beam monitoring and dosimetry techniques capable of sustaining very-high-dose rates are developed. Last, but not least, software tools for FLASH treatment planning are also needed to evaluate the technique's potential and to enable clinical applications.

FLASH effect has been observed using electron, photon, and proton beams [10–13], but the use of electron beams seems to represent the most viable and cost-effective solution to clinical applications, due to the recent improvement of electron linear accelerator technology [14]. As far as X-ray beams are concerned, the anode of an X-ray tube should meet the requirements of resisting the enormous instantaneous power asked by FLASH RT applications, without melting or being damaged. If we consider instead a few MeV external RT photons, produced from linac that already proved to be capable of reaching FLASH intensities, we see that the achievable intensity is limited by the photons production mechanism, occurring via the Bremsstrahlung effect, which greatly reduces the final beam intensity. Providing photon beams of the required intensity in a clinical environment via this technique is, therefore, a challenge that has yet to be addressed. Concerning protons, indeed, the technical challenge is currently the development of an ultra-fast pencil beam scanning technique capable of fully covering the target volume at the high-dose rates needed by FLASH RT applications.

For these reasons, currently, electron FLASH RT is the logical first choice to be investigated for the transition from preclinical research to the first clinical applications. In particular, the use of monoenergetic high-intensity pulses of electrons of 9–12 MeV energy makes intraoperative radiotherapy (IOeRT) the current best candidate for translation to the clinic.

In this context, another field that is experiencing a renewed interest is related to EBRT performed using electrons of energies in the 50–200 MeV range. The clinical implementation of such very high energy electrons (VHEE) as a solution for EBRT has been pursued in the past but with several difficulties related to the high complexity of the system needed to fit the VHEE accelerator inside the treatment room and to the specific features of the interaction of the electron with the patient tissues. Electron beams suffer more than proton beams from the broadening due to multiple scattering interactions in the patient's body and for that reason, very-high energies are needed to ensure that the organs at risk (OAR) close to the tumor are properly spared. For that very last reason, the sparing potential that occurs in the FLASH irradiation could ease the VHEE use in EBRT allowing to overcome all the difficulties that prevented the spreading of this technique.

4.2 State of the Art of FLASH Radiotherapy

The FLASH effect polarized the attention of the scientific community in RT since its discovery in 2014 when it was shown that ultra-fast radiation reduces toxicity in healthy tissues while keeping an efficient control of the tumor as in the conventional RT. In the first FLASH experiment, mice were irradiated both in conventional (CONV) and FLASH modality. FLASH irradiation was performed using an electron linac with a nominal energy of 5.6 MeV. The delivered dose was

17 Gy in CONV and FLASH modalities with large differences in the mean dose rate: 0.03 Gy/s and 60 Gy/s, respectively. The outcome of this study revealed that FLASH irradiation avoided radiation-induced fibrosis in lungs but kept CONV irradiation efficiency in the control of tumor growth. The FLASH effect was confirmed in larger mammals by M.C. Vozenin et al. who performed a dose escalation study on the skin response in a mini-pig model [2]. The irradiation was performed with doses ranging from 22 to 34 Gy on the same animal and a mean dose rate ranging from 0.1 to 340 Gy/s with instantaneous dose rates reaching 1.9×10^6 Gy/s. The radiation-induced fibro-necrosis was observed after 32 weeks in the conventional dose rate exposures at doses of 28–31–34 Gy; whereas, no skin reaction was observed with FLASH-RT at similar doses. Thirty-six weeks post radiotherapy, the necrosis lesions visible in conventional irradiated spots were absent in FLASH-irradiated spots. The FLASH-RT translation to the clinic has already started [5]. The first patient treatment was carried out in Lausanne Hospital: The patient was a 75-year-old man with a multi-resistant CD30+ T-cell cutaneous lymphoma on the skin surface. The tumor was irradiated with 6 MeV electrons dedicated linac using 15 Gy with a mean dose rate of 166 Gy/s and an instantaneous dose rate equal to 1.5×10^6. After a follow-up of 5 months, the patient showed complete tumor regression.

A large number of in vivo radiobiological experiments recorded significant normal tissue sparing using electron irradiation at ultra-high-dose rates across various species such as small rodents (mice) [15, 16] and developing organisms [17], and on different clinical endpoints as lung fibrosis [4], neurocognitive impairment [3], developmental disorder and deformity [16], severe skin reactions [18], and gastrointestinal syndrome [16], but the underlying radiobiological basis of the FLASH effect remains to be fully understood.

4.2.1 FLASH Parameters

The definition of the FLASH regime requires the specification of different interdependent temporal parameters such as pulse repetition frequency (PRF) (i.e., the time between two subsequent pulses), pulse number n_p and pulse width t_p (time window length of each radiation pulse), dose per pulse (D_p), in-peak dose rate, as well as the time-averaged dose rate and the total irradiation time from the first to the last delivered pulses.

Currently, there is still an intense ongoing research activity to experimentally characterize these parameters, but the scientific community, based on low-energy radiobiological experiments, has reached a consensus on some reference values needed for the FLASH effect to occur. In particular, the total irradiation time should be kept under 100 ms [19] with mean dose rates above 100 Gy/s [3] and instantaneous dose rates of 10^6 Gy/s or more. In addition, a single pulse must deliver at least 1–2 Gy, three orders of magnitude higher than the dose per pulse of a conventional medical linac (1 mGy/pulse), whereby the pulse duration is comparable (few μs). These FLASH parameters are illustrated in Fig. 4.2 and their reference values are given in Table 4.1.

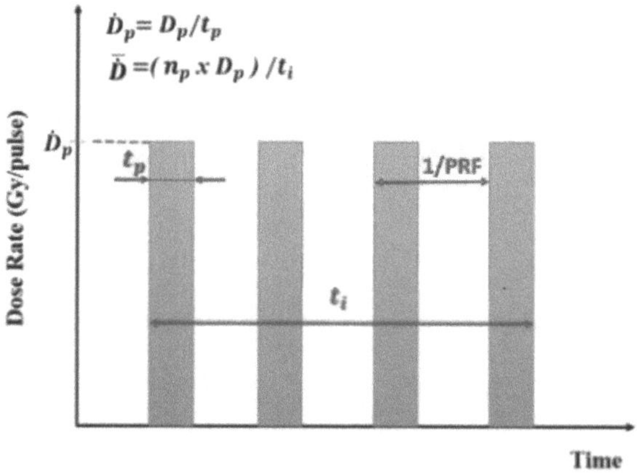

Figure 4.2 Scheme of a pulsed beam temporal structure.

Table 4.1 Most used parameters for FLASH irradiation

Symbol	Description	Value
PRF	Pulse repetition frequency	> 100 Hz
t_p	Pulse width	0.1–4.0 μs
t_i	Total irradiation time	< 100 ms
$D^{\cdot}$	Time-averaged dose rate	> 100 Gy/s
Dp	Dose-rate in a single pulse	> 10^6 Gy/s
D_p	Dose in a single pulse	> 1 Gy

4.2.2 Beam Monitoring and Dosimetry in FLASH Therapy

Beam monitoring is essential to keep under control the accelerator performances during irradiation, so as to secure the precision required for quality assurance (QA) and to allow a rapid and reliable system for machine tuning. Furthermore, online dosimetry during radiotherapy is essential for patient safety, treatment precision, and effectiveness in reaching the tumor target. This contributes to maximizing therapeutic outcomes and minimizing side effects.

Since the FLASH effect is strongly related to the high-dose rate in a single pulse and the total dose delivered over the treated volume, it is crucial to have online access to dose and beam position during irradiation. This poses an unprecedented technical challenge, since most devices currently used in the standard RT treatment suffer from irradiation rate-dependent effects. The ionization chamber (IC), the most popular device for online dosimetry in clinical use, saturates when exposed to FLASH intensity. The IC response becomes non-linear with the delivered dose; therefore, its ability to accurately measure the dose is compromised. As a consequence, specifically designed ionization chambers are needed to deal with the high-dose rates regime, ensuring a linear response and accuracy in measurements.

Alternative methods or technologies must be explored to overcome the limitations associated with traditional devices. Among the explored choices for real-time measurements, scintillation-based and solid-state detectors (in particular diamonds) have shown good linearity of the response with increasing dose rates [20].

There are also several non-real-time dosimeters used to measure dose in FLASH regimes. Some of these include Gafchromic films, alanine dosimeters, and diode dosimeters.

Gafchromic films change color in response to exposure to ionizing radiation. They can be used to measure the total dose received during a FLASH treatment; however, the reading is performed after the treatment. Alanine dosimeters are devices based on the paramagnetic resonance of electrons in the alanine molecule. These dosimeters can be used to measure the total absorbed dose during FLASH treatment. Like Gafchromic films, the reading of alanine dosimeters occurs post-treatment. Diodes are commonly used to measure dose in conventional radiotherapy. They can also be applied to assess dose in FLASH regimes, but the reading takes place after exposure. It is important to note that even if these dosimeters do not provide real-time information during FLASH treatment, they are still crucial for evaluating and verifying the total dose distribution received in these high-dose-rate treatments.

4.2.3 Characterization of Ultra-High-Dose Rate with Gafchromic Films

Gafchromic films have a relevant role in dose measurements and beam monitoring, especially in the context of FLASH irradiation. When it comes to beam monitoring, these films can be used to measure the percentage depth dose (PDD) distribution and the transverse profile of the beam.

The PDD distribution describes the percentage distribution of the dose deposition along the beam path and provides fundamental information like the shape and the maximum of the dose delivery.

In the following, as an example, we show the results of a campaign of measurements on a FLASH linac performed at Institute Curie (Orsay, France).

The main beam parameters are reported in Table 4.2. The nominal output electron beam energies are 5 MeV and 7 MeV, and the electron pulses, with peak currents of up to 120 mA, have an adjustable RF pulse duration between 0.5 and 4 μs. The electron beam parameters allow irradiation in conventional and FLASH modes. In conventional mode, online dosimetry makes use of two ionization chambers that are automatically removed from the beam axis when the FLASH regime is selected. The beam current, in the case of FLASH mode, can be measured using a pair of induction toroids.

Table 4.2 Main features of electron FLASH

Parameter	Value
Output energy	5 or 7 MeV
Pulse repetition frequency	1–250 Hz
Pulse width	0.5–4 μs
Maximum peak beam current 7 MeV	120 mA
Maximum peak beam current 5 MeV	108 mA

For the measurements, hollow PMMA cylinders, made of polymethyl methacrylate, with 30 mm or 120 mm inner diameters were positioned aligned with the beam axis, between the radiation source and the target area to shape the radiation field. Gafchromic films, specifically EBT-XD (Ashland Inc., Wilmington, DE, USA), were employed in a PMMA slab phantom to explore PDD and beam transverse profiles at various depths. For PDD FLASH measurements, films were positioned parallel to the beam axis in the PMMA phantom and irradiated with 7 MeV beams using applicators A-d120 and A-d30, with a pulse width of 4 μs. Additionally, three films were irradiated at the dose peak value depth (R100), 80% depth (R80), and 50% depth (R50). Twenty-four hours post-irradiation, the films were scanned using an Epson 800, 48-bit color scanner, and the dose maps were analyzed using FilmQA Pro software [25], employing triple-channel and reference dose protocols. The comparison of the experimental measurements with the MC simulations obtained using 2020.0.10 FLUKA, as shown in Fig. 4.3.

The results of dose measurements conducted with Gafchromic films at the R100 point, utilizing the previously described applicators (A-d30 and A-d120) at 7 MeV with a maximum pulse width of 4 μs, are presented in Table 4.3. The uncertainty associated with EBT-XD dose determination is within ±5%.

Table 4.3 Dose per pulse achievable with a different applicator at 4 μs pulse duration

Applicator size ø [mm]	7 MeV dose per pulse at 4 μs [Gy]
120	3
30	19

All of these measurements related to the PDD and the transverse profile of the beam were conducted under the FLASH regime. In fact, for the 30 mm applicator, the maximum delivered dose was 19 Gy, while for the 12 cm applicator, it was 3 Gy. Since we consistently use the same current, irradiating two vastly different areas results in distinct doses per pulse. As depicted in Fig 4.4, the beam profiles exhibit remarkable homogeneity.

The homogeneity and reproducibility of measurements of PDD and beam profiles obtained with Gafchromic films make these devices particularly suitable for dosimetry in the FLASH radiation regime.

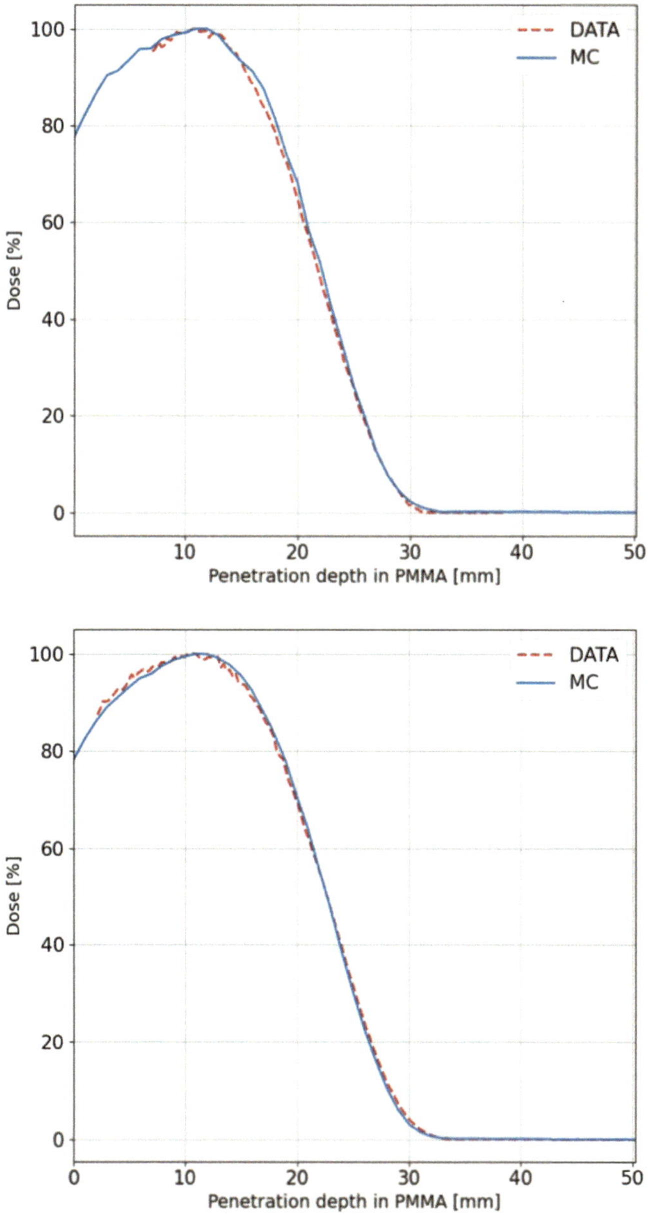

Figure 4.3 Measured (dotted red line) and simulated (blue line) PDD in PMMA phantom obtained for the 7 MeV electrons beam collimated with the A-d30 (top) and A-d120 (bottom) applicators [8].

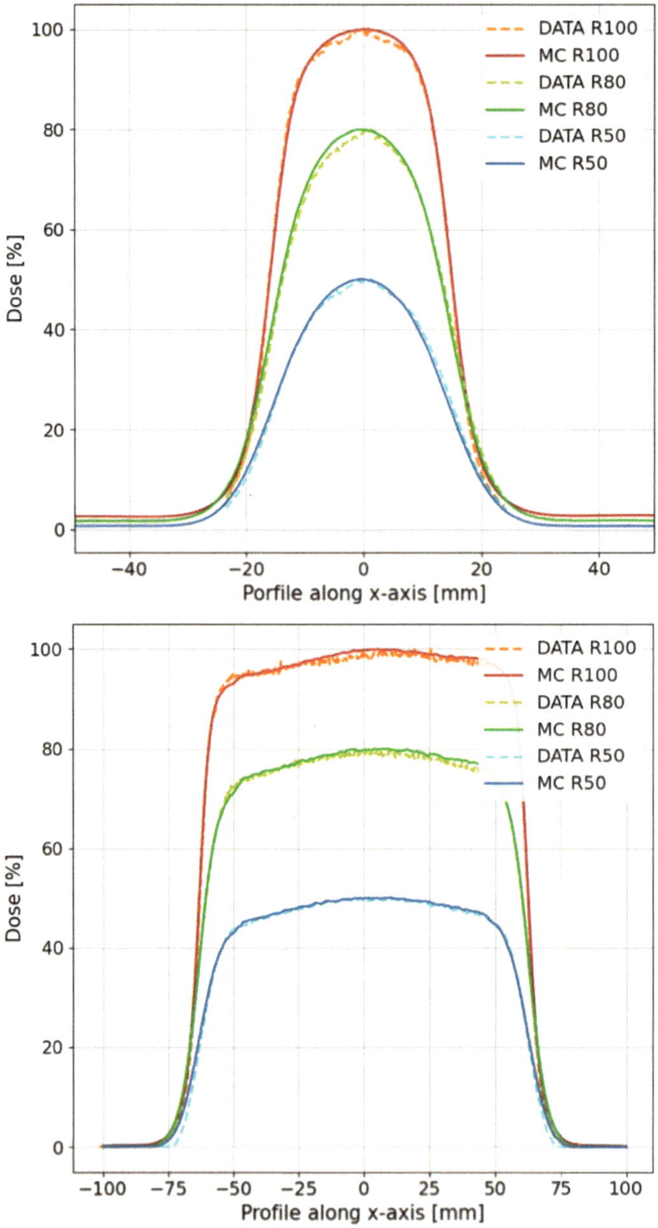

Figure 4.4 Measured (dotted line) and simulated (continuous line) transverse profile in the PMMA phantom obtained for the 7 MeV electrons beam collimated with the A-d30 (top) and A-d120 (bottom) applicators. The figures show the profiles obtained at 13 mm (R100), 17 mm (R80), and 21 mm (R50) depth [8].

4.2.4 New Detectors for Ultra-High-Dose Rate Irradiation

Passive dosimeters, like alanine and Gafchromic films, have proven effective for specific applications despite inherent limitations. A remarkable drawback is the delayed response. Since it can take even hours or days after the irradiation to have the dose measurement results, this makes these detectors unfit for daily linac quality assurance and online measurements. Several research groups are developing real-time detectors to provide PDD in the FLASH regime. A typical example is the FLASH diamond (FD), a diamond Schottky diode detector designed specifically for ultra-high dose per pulse (UH-DPP) and UH-DR applications. Rigorous characterization has validated the FD's response linearity for dose per pulse (DPP) values up to 20 Gy, average dose rates of about 1 kGy/s, and instantaneous dose rates of approximately 5 MGy/s, establishing its viability for FLASH-RT applications. Must be stressed that calibrated diamond detectors can serve as reliable reference dosimeters, due to their very high response stability.

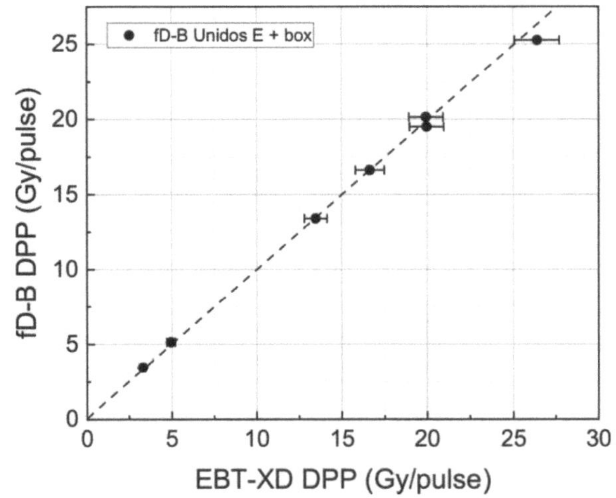

Figure 4.5 Dose per pulse measured by the FD at the Curie Institute. The plot shows a linear response of the detector with respect to the GAF-chromic measurements [20].

As an example, we present the outcomes of a measurement campaign conducted on a FLASH linac at the Institute Curie (Orsay, France). The characterization of diamond prototypes under ultra-high DPP irradiation conditions was made using electron beams generated by electron FLASH linac. Under typical irradiation conditions, DPPs of approximately 10 Gy/s can be achieved, resulting in instantaneous dose rates of several MGy/s and average dose rates of around 1 kGy/s. The response of an FD is shown in Fig. 4.5 with respect to the Gafchromic film results (EBT-XD model). The comparison of the measurement was evaluated up to DPP values of 26 Gy/pulse. The dashed line in the plot represents the perfect correspondence between diamond and film measurement. In the GAF measurement, a 5% uncertainty has been taken into account.

An indirect confirmation of the stability of FD response is provided by the measurements of dose distributions (PDDs) obtained in three different setup conditions, as shown in Fig 4.6, up to at least 20 Gy/pulse. These results provide clear evidence of the suitability of a diamond detector for FLASH-RT applications.

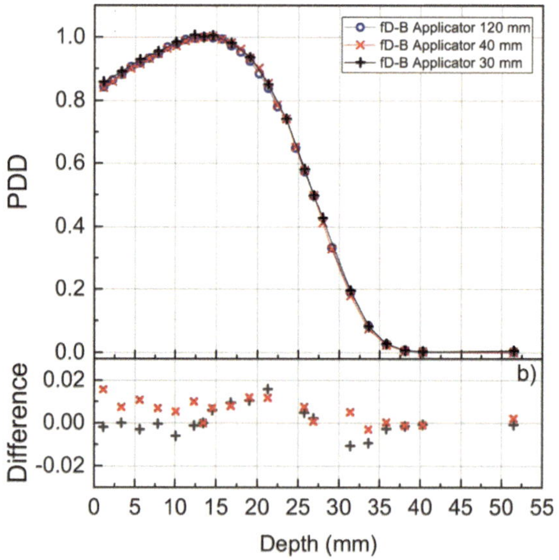

Figure 4.6 Percentage depth dose measurements by the FD-B prototype at Curie Institute. The three datasets refer to the measurements performed by using the 120-, 40-, and 30-mm applicators [20].

4.3 VHEE FLASH-RT

Electrons of high energy never reached the clinical implementation stage. As a consequence, the software for a dedicated treatment planning system (TPS) for treatments delivered using VHEE is not commercially available. For this reason, there is current effort, both in academic institutions and industrial companies, to develop such software tools that are needed to define each beam direction, energy, intensity, and angular spread to deliver the prescribed dose to the PTV while achieving the best sparing of the surrounding OARs.

Such a planning software can also be used to evaluate the effective VHEE FLASH potential against other state-of-the-art EBRT technologies like photon intensity-modulated radiotherapy (IMRT), photon volumetric modulated arc therapy (VMAT), or proton beam treatment to have a reliable estimation of the VHEE potential with respect to existing RT technologies.

The treatment of deep-seated tumors exploiting electrons of energy in the 50–250 MeV range has been already explored in the past [21, 22]. From the physical point of view, the dose release of electrons represents a compromise between protons and photons. Being lighter than protons, they exhibit a broader Bragg peak (BP). However, being charged particles, they suffer from multiple scattering interactions, unlike photons, resulting in a less conformal lateral dose release (see Fig. 4.7).

Also, VHEE can be delivered at FLASH rates, with respect to the low-energy electrons used in eIORT a VHEE linac requires a further acceleration stage, which usually does not have a disrupting effect on the transported current. An appealing feature of VHEE is the small magnetic rigidity compared to protons, which allows easier magnetic bending of the beam when delivered in an active scanning, pencil beams approach. The broader PDD of VHEE does not have the selectivity potential of other RT-charged beams as proton or carbon, but allows to overcome two main limitations of UHDR irradiation with hadrons. There is no need to change the beam energy to cover a large target volume (electrons provide a naturally spread-out BP), and this greatly helps in providing the required a high-dose rate, and there is no need to implement strict safety margins on the patient positioning as the longitudinal absorbed dose distribution does not exhibit any sharp fall.

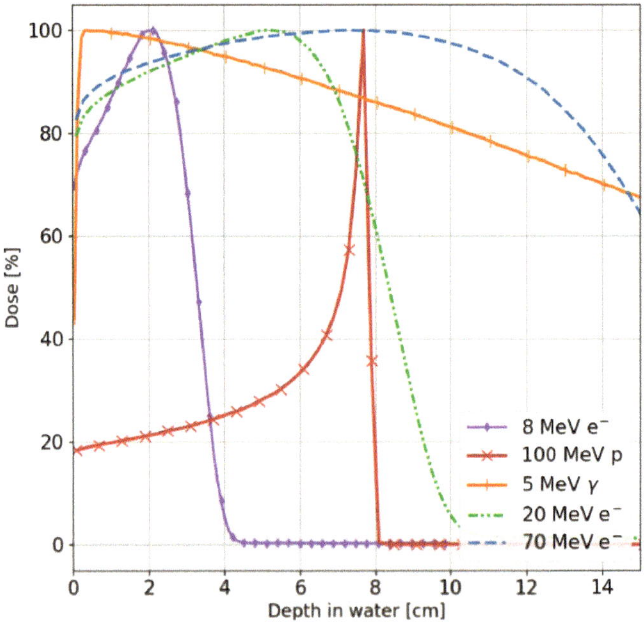

Figure 4.7 Percentage dose profiles along the beam axis for 8 MeV (violet line), 20 MeV (green line), and 70 MeV (blue line) electrons, 5 MeV photons (orange line), and 100 MeV protons (red line) in a water phantom obtained using FRED Monte Carlo software [23–25].

The FLASH effect might also mitigate the need for very high energies. While it has already been shown [21, 22] that VHEE is competitive with protons and conventional RT at energies above 150 MeV, the UHDR beam delivery might allow for improved OARs sparing even in the case of lower energy electron beams.

To evaluate the FLASH VHEE irradiation performances in clinical conditions both the dose and the dose rate have to be considered in the TPS and the dose release optimization must be performed taking into account the FLASH conditions request. While the evaluation of the absorbed dose can now be carried out with great precision using Monte Carlo (MC) simulations, such as FLUKA [26], GEANT4 [27], or FRED [23–25] MC, the dose rate evaluation requires some additional inputs. In particular, the dose rate is dependent on the PTV coverage strategy and on the detail of the specific beam delivery system of the VHEE linac.

4.3.1 FLASH-VHEE Therapy Potential

Assuming as baseline VHEE machine, an RF linac that is an evolution of the current eIORT FLASH electron system, the main VHEE FLASH delivery features will be short (few μs) pulses, with a pulse repetition frequency ranging from 100 Hz to 1 kHz, achieving instantaneous dose rates several orders of magnitude larger than the ones required to trigger the FLASH effect.

In this landscape, to evaluate the FLASH potential in cancer treatments and thus quantify the reduced radiation-induced toxicity in normal tissues, a preliminary FLASH-modifying factor (FMF) is introduced when compared to conventional treatments. The FMF is defined as the ratio of doses that need to be administered at conventional dose rates (D_{CONV}) and UHDR (D_{UHDR}) to achieve an isoeffect for a given biological system and endpoint [28]:

$$\mathrm{FMF} = \frac{D_{\mathrm{CONV}}}{D_{\mathrm{UHDR}_{\mathrm{isoeffect}}}} \tag{4.1}$$

An FMF value lower than 1 represents the normal tissue-sparing effect of UHDR compared to conventional irradiation, and therefore, the normal tissue-sparing by the FLASH effect increases as the FMF decreases. Utilizing this concept, a dose D delivered with UHDR can be converted as follows into an isoeffective FMF-weighted dose D_{FMF} delivered at conventional dose rates:

$$D_{\mathrm{FMF}} = \mathrm{FMF} \cdot D \tag{4.2}$$

Experimental in vivo data show that the magnitude of the FMF generally decreases (indicating increased sparing) as a function of the single-fraction dose. The analysis revealed that individual data series can be effectively described by a piece-wise linear function [28]:

$$\mathrm{FMF}(D_{\mathrm{FMF}^{\min},D_{\mathrm{Th}}}) = \frac{1}{(1-\mathrm{FMF}^{\min})\frac{D_{\mathrm{Th}}}{D} + \mathrm{FMF}^{\min}} \quad \begin{matrix} \mathit{for}\ D \le D_{\mathrm{T}} \\ \mathit{for}\ D > D_{\mathrm{T}} \end{matrix} \tag{4.3}$$

Here, D represents the absorbed dose, D_{Th} denotes the minimum threshold dose required for the occurrence of the FLASH effect, and $\mathrm{FMF}^{\min}$ stands for the minimum attainable FMF value. This behavior

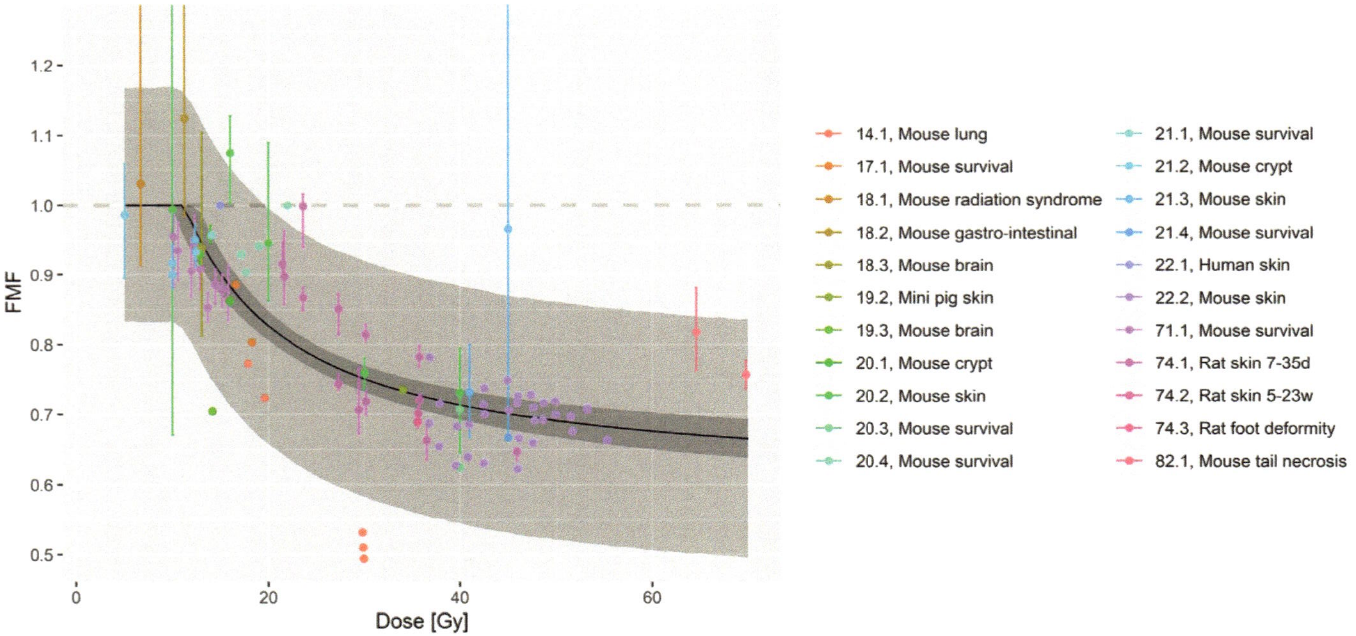

Figure 4.8 Pooled mammalian data plotted as FLASH-modifying factor (FMF) versus single-fraction ultra-high-dose rate dose. A regression to the data using the sudden effect transition (SET) function is shown (solid line) with the 95% prediction interval (light gray band) and 95% confidence interval (dark gray band) [28].

corresponds to a sudden effect transition (SET), which is consistent with any phenomenon causing the radiobiological effectiveness of the deposited dose beyond D_{Th} to abruptly shift from 1 to a reduced constant value of $\mathrm{FMF}^{\mathrm{min}}$, where $\mathrm{FMF}^{\mathrm{min}}$ is less than 1.

Figure 4.8 displays selected data series from individual experiments, each including four or more data points. The plot illustrates the relationship between D_{FMF} and the single fraction dose D. A consistent trend is observed along most of the collected data samples with FMF values decreasing monotonically for larger doses, with the exception of those related to mouse skin. It is worth noticing that many of these FMF values exhibit significant uncertainties and, in general, all the data are quite scattered around the average behavior.

The existence of the SET effect shows that the FLASH gain is maximized in highly hypofractionated treatment in which the dose per fraction ranges between 6 and 10 Gy (possible for instance in prostate, pancreas, and lung cancer). However, care has to be taken in balancing the OARs sparing achieved with UHDR irradiation at a high fraction dose with possible increased toxicity induced in the OARs due to the high dose itself.

4.3.2 The Case of Pancreatic Cancer

Using an FMF-based modeling of the FLASH effect, it is possible to explore, using analytical representation or MC simulations of the dose release, the impact of FLASH irradiation.

We report here, as an example, a real case of pancreatic cancer, in which a hypofractionated approach is usually chosen. The patient underwent stereotactic body radiation therapy with a high dose per fraction (6 Gy) at Campus Biomedico Hospital, Rome, Italy, with volumetric modulated arc therapy (VMAT) with photons.

The simulation of a possible VHEE treatment required CT information, the geometry of the beam directions focusing on the patient (fields), and the specification of the transverse setup of the fields, while the FRED MC software was used to calculate the absorbed dose maps. An intensity-modulated radiation therapy (IMRT)-like configuration with seven static fields was used following preliminary work performed on prostate cancer [29] and intracranial lesions [30]. The simulated electron pencil beams had a transverse size of a few mm and a divergence of mrad. The analysis was limited to the 70–130 MeV energy range, assuming an active scanning-like beam delivery technology.

Once absorbed dose maps were obtained for each pencil beam foreseen in the treatment plan, all the pencil beam fluences were optimized to achieve the required coverage of the PTV while sparing OARs. A widely used tool to evaluate an RT treatment is the dose volume histograms (DHV). In a DVH, the fraction of a tissue volume (tumor, OAR) is plotted versus the fraction of the prescribed dose given to that specific volume fraction.

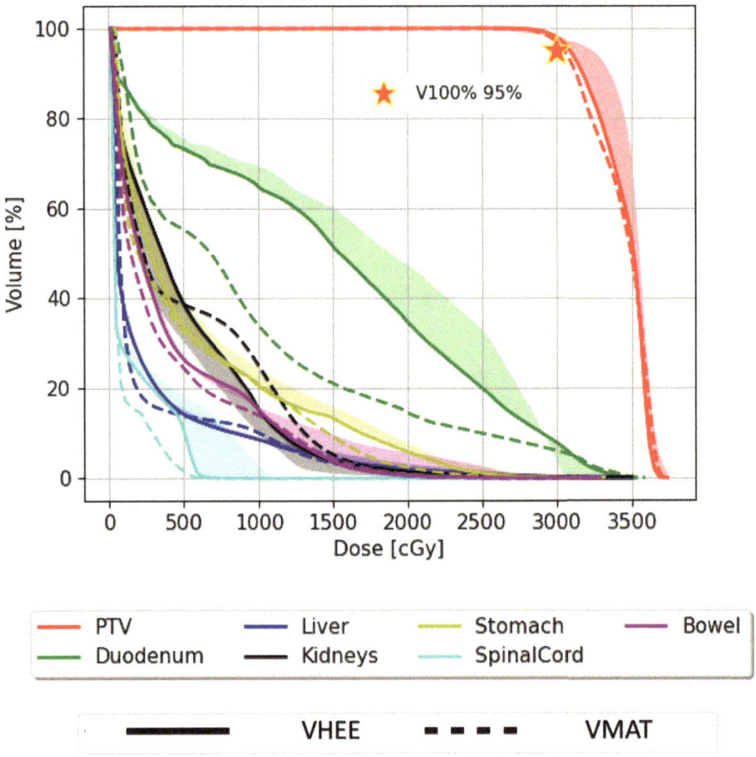

Figure 4.9 DVHs for the PTV and main OARs obtained from the delivered VMAT plan (dashed line) and the simulated VHEE one (solid line). The transparent bands indicate the potential improvement achievable if the plan is delivered with an ultra-high-dose rate (UHDR). These bands span from the best-case scenario, where the $FMF^{min} = 0.6$ and $D_{Th} = 5$ Gy, to the worst-case scenario with no additional sparing effect. The best-case scenario was obtained by optimizing the biological dose D_{FMF} evaluated as reported in Ref. [28].

Figure 4.9 shows the DVH as an example in the study. It can be seen that VMAT (dashed line) and VHEE (solid line) plans have comparable quality, with one important detail in favor of VHEE. The use of VHEE allows for a significant improvement in PTV coverage while keeping the dose delivered to the duodenum within the optimal constraint for this organ and all other organs at risk. The transparent bands represent the curves corresponding to the different FLASH plans, in which the biological dose D_{FMF} was computed and optimized according to different FMF and dose thresholds assumed for the FLASH effect. From the figure, it is evident that FLASH optimization leads to an increase in the absorbed dose by the PTV, while simultaneously reducing the maximum dose absorbed by critical OARs once the set threshold dose in the model is exceeded (D_{Th} = 5 Gy per fraction).

4.4 Electron Linear Accelerator for FLASH Radiotherapy

The FLASH effect was observed also with photons and protons but so far most of the pre-clinical studies investigating the FLASH effect used electron beams generated by dedicated or modified linacs. Furthermore, the clinical implementation of the FLASH effect is very likely to be first introduced in intraoperative RT or the treatment of dermatologic tumors. Both these treatments can be done with an electron beam of energies in the 7–12 MeV. The low-energy electron linacs are then devices of large interest for the FLASH effect application.

The Kinetron [31] and Oriatron eRT6 [7] electron linacs, at Orsay and Lausanne University Hospital, respectively, are nowadays the most recognizable FLASH sources in the current literature, used for the successful in vivo treatments of small animals and a single patient. The Kinetron is now decommissioned, and it has been replaced by the electron FLASH (EF) [32], which generates electron beams of 5–7 MeV, with a peak current of 100 mA. The Oriatron eRT6 allows the control of the energy from 4.9 to 6 MeV, with PRF from 5 to 200 Hz, and pulse width from 0.5 to 2.2 μs. Moreover, the triode electron gun grid tension (0–300 V) can drive a peak beam current of up to 300 mA.

4.4.1 Low-Energy Linac

Typically, a linear accelerator (linac) designed for low-energy (5–9 MeV) radiotherapy irradiation includes a thermionic gun, a modulator, a magnetron, a circulator, and an accelerating structure. Figure 4.10 illustrates a schematic representation of the principal components of an S-band (2.998 GHz) FLASH linac, focusing on the crucial elements of the accelerator. The electron beam is generated by a thermionic electron gun, where electrons are emitted from the surface of a cathode, heated to several hundred degrees Celsius by a low-voltage current in a filament. The linac is powered by a radiofrequency source, typically a magnetron. To prevent reflections from the linac to the magnetron, which could potentially damage it, a circulator is strategically installed between the two devices. The circulator, a passive non-reciprocal device with three or more ports, is aimed to isolate the RF power sources from microwave power back reflected, both at the beginning and end of each RF pulse.

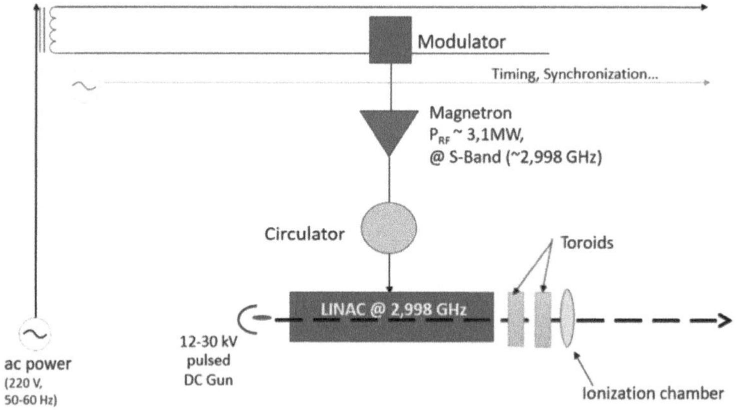

Figure 4.10 Main medical linac components scheme.

The described linac configuration needs a pulse modulator to generate high-power pulses characterized by a rapid rise time, a flat top, and short duration, essential to drive a high-power magnetron.

A FLASH linac differs from a conventional medical linac, in that, it is designed to deliver a higher dose in shorter times and, therefore, must be able to accelerate a large number of charges, typically of the order of hundreds of nano coulombs (nC), in a single pulse.

This figure must be compared to the pico coulombs (pC) amount of accelerated charge of the conventional case.

4.4.2 VHEE Linac

The key advantage of a VHEE beam over a conventional photon beam is the possibility to achieve a better dose conformality with the possibility to reach easily a FLASH regime with a setup that is comparable in cost and size. The comparison of the VHEE option with the proton RT underlines the potential to have a clinical accelerator at considerably reduced costs compared to what is currently necessary for a proton beam installation. This makes VHEE beams an intriguing and potentially cost-effective alternative for cancer treatment.

Different technological solutions have been adopted [33] for the design of the VHEE machine, depending on the operating resonant frequency, which represents one of the most RF-relevant parameters to choose when designing a linac. Scaling laws indicate that, as the frequency of RF cavities increases, it becomes possible to achieve the needed beam energy with a shorter accelerator length for a given power. In the past, significant progress was made in the development of warm X-band traveling wave (TW) structures, achieving an accelerating gradient of 100 MV/m [34–36]. These X-band developments were mainly driven by the need for future accelerators for high-energy physics. More recently, C-band warm TW structures achieved a gradient of 50 MV/m [37–40] and have been mainly used in free electron laser and Compton sources.

In this scenario, the Sapienza University of Rome and the Italian Institute of Nuclear Physics (INFN) proposed a new project, whose schematic representation is shown in Fig. 4.11.

It consists of one standing wave injector and two traveling wave high-gradient accelerating structures operating at a working frequency of 5.712 GHz with the C-band technology that offers a compact design. The standing wave (SW) injector is capable of accelerating the current emitted from a pulsed DC gun to an energy of 10 MeV. Subsequently, the beam is directed into two consecutive linear traveling wave (TW) structures, each 1 meter long, featuring a high accelerating gradient. The three structures are intended to be powered by a single 50 MW Klystron, providing an effective available power of 45 MW.

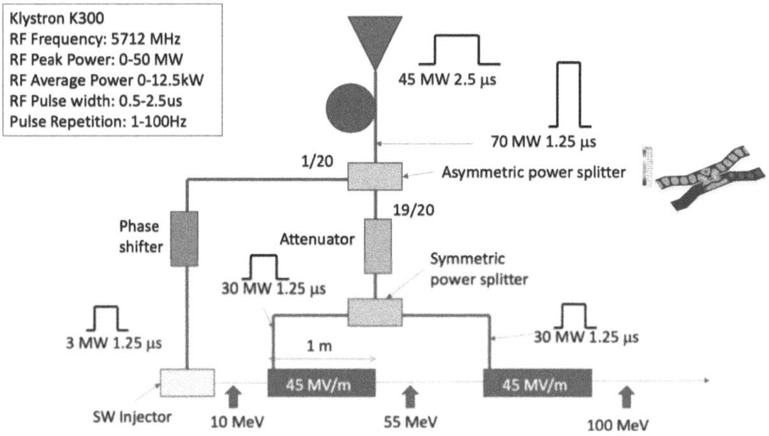

Figure 4.11 Basic layout of the Sapienza–INFN project.

In conclusion, the C band linac presented here can accelerate FLASH beams, with a high dose per pulse and dose rate, in the range of 50–100 MeV in about 3 mt. This machine design, for its compactness, relatively low cost, and high-dose-rate performances, could be the perfect option for a viable VHEE machine with FLASH capability to be translated into clinical practice.

4.5 Conclusions

FLASH radiation therapy stands at the forefront of advancements in cancer radiation therapy, showing significant promise in both preclinical and clinical research. The momentum gained in this research area is evident in the initiatives undertaken by several universities and research institutions. A huge research effort on FLASH therapy focused on understanding the basic mechanisms underlying FLASH biological effects and its radiobiology, in particular, to assess its impact on tumor cells and surrounding healthy tissues.

At the same time, to support the translation in clinical practice, researchers are also working on optimizing the treatment protocols for FLASH therapy. This includes refining the timing, dosage, and frequency of treatments to maximize therapeutic benefits while minimizing potential side effects.

However, no implementation of this new RT technique would be possible without a robust enhancement of the beam delivery techniques. In this field, ongoing efforts are focused on technical innovations and on developing compact solutions for machines capable of delivering the ultra-high-dose rate needed by FLASH RT. Furthermore, significant endeavors are currently being directed toward dosimetry, beam monitoring, beam delivery, and treatment planning.

By addressing these diverse aspects of research, the scientific community aims to comprehensively advance FLASH therapy toward becoming a well-established and effective option in cancer treatment.

References

1. A. Schüller, S. Heinrich, C. Fouillade, A. Subiel, L. De Marzi, F. Romano, P. Peier, M. Trachsel, C. Fleta, R. Kranzer, M. Caresana, S. Salvador, S. Busold, A. Schönfeld, M. McEwen, F. Gomez, J. Solc, C. Bailat, V. Linhart, J. Jakubek, J. Pawelke, M. Borghesi, R.-P. Kapsch, A. Knyziak, A. Boso, V. Olsovcova, C. Kottler, D. Poppinga, I. Ambrozova, C.-S. Schmitzer, S. Rossomme, M.-C. Vozenin. The European joint research project UHD pulse – metrology for advanced radiotherapy using particle beams with ultra-high pulse dose rates, *Physica Medica,* 80, 2020, 134–150. https://doi.org/10.1016/j.ejmp.2020.09.020.
2. M. Vozenin, P. De Fornel, K. Petersson, et al. The advantage of FLASH radiotherapy confirmed in mini-pig and cat cancer patients, *Clin. Cancer. Res.,* 25, 2018, 35–42. doi: 10.1158/1078- 0432.CCR-17-3375.
3. K. Montay-Gruel, M. Petersson, M. Jaccard, et al. Irradiation in a FLASH: Unique sparing of memory in mice after whole brain irradiation with dose rates above 100 Gy/s, *Radiother. Oncol.,* 124, 2017, 365–369. doi: 10.1016/j.radonc.2017.05.003.
4. C. Fouillade, S. Curras-Alonso, L. Giuranno, E. Quelennec, S. Heinrich, S. Bonnet-Boissinot, A. Beddok, S. Leboucher, H. U. Karakurt, M. Bohec, et al. Flash irradiation spares lung progenitor cells and limits the incidence of radio-induced senescence FLASH-RT spares lung progenitor cells, *Clinical Cancer Research,* 26 (6), 2020, 1497–1506.

5. J. Bourhis, W. Sozzi, P. Gon¸calves Jorge, et al. Treatment of a first patient with FLASH-radiotherapy, *Radiother. Oncol.*, 139, 2019, 18–22. doi: 10.1016/j.radonc.2019.06.019.
6. R. Moeckli, P. Gonçalves Jorge, V. Griljand, et al. Commissioning of an ultra-high dose rate pulsed electron beam medical LINAC for FLASH RT preclinical animal experiments and future clinical human protocols, *Med. Phys.*, 48 (6), 2021, 3134–3139.
7. M. Jaccard, M. Durán, K. Petersson, et al. High dose-per-pulse electron beam dosimetry: Commissioning of the Oriatron eRT6 prototype linear accelerator for preclinical use, *Med Phys.*, 45 (2), 2018, 863–874.
8. L. Giuliano, G. Franciosini, L. Palumbo, L. Aggar, M. Dutreix, L. Faillace, V. Favaudon, G. Felici, F. Galante, A. Mostacci, M. Migliorati, M. Pacitti, A. Patriarca, S. Heinrich. Characterization of ultra-high-dose rate electron beams with electron flash linac, *Applied Sciences*, 13 (1), 2023. doi: 10.3390/app13010631.
9. K. Petersson, M. Jaccard, J.-F. Germond, T. Buchillier, F. Bochud, J. Bourhis, M.-C. Vozenin, C. Bailat. High dose-per-pulse electron beam dosimetry — a model to correct for the ion recombination in the advanced Markus ionization chamber, *Medical Physics*, 44 (3), 2017, 1157–1167. arXiv: https://aapm.onlinelibrary.wiley.com/doi/pdf/10.1002/mp.12111, doi: https://doi.org/10.1002/mp.12111.
10. V. Favaudon, L. Caplier, V. Monceau, F. Pouzoulet, M. Sayarath, C. Fouillade, M.- F. Poupon, I. Brito, P. Hupé, J. Bourhis, J. Hall, J.-J. Fontaine, M.-C. Vozenin. Ultrahigh dose-rate flash irradiation increases the differential response between normal and tumor tissue in mice, *Science Translational Medicine*, 6 (245), 2014, 245ra93–245ra93. a r X i v : https://www.science.org/doi/pdf/10.1126/scitranslmed.3008973, doi: 10.1126/scitranslmed.3008973.
11. P. Montay-Gruel, et al. Flash radiotherapy with photon beams, *Medical Physics,* 2021. arXiv: https://aapm.onlinelibrary.wiley.com/doi/pdf/10.1002/mp.15222, https://doi.org/10.1002/mp.15222.
12. M. G. Ronga, et al. Back to the future: Very high-energy electrons (VHEEs) and their potential application in radiation therapy, *Cancers,* 13 (19), 2021). doi: 10.3390/cancers13194942.
13. E. S. Diffenderfer, et al. Design, implementation, and in vivo validation of a novel proton flash radiation therapy system, *International Journal of Radiation Oncology Biology Physics,* 106 (2), 2020, 440–448. https://doi.org/10.1016/j.ijrobp.2019.10.049.

14. L. Faillace, et al. Compact S-band linear accelerator system for ultrafast, ultrahigh dose-rate radiotherapy, *Phys. Rev. Accel. Beams,* 24, 2021, 050102. doi: 10.1103/PhysRevAccelBeams.24.050102.

15. J. H. Hendry, J. V. Moore, B. W. Hodgson, J. P. Keene. The constant low oxygen concentration in all the target cells for mouse tail radio necrosis, *Radiation Research,* 92 (1), 1982, 172–181.

16. E. Schueler, S. Trovati, G. King, F. Lartey, M. Rafat, B. Loo, P. Maxim. Tu-h-campus-tep2-02: Flash irradiation improves the therapeutic index following GI tract irradiation, *Medical Physics,* 43 (6Part37), 2016, 3783–3783. arXiv: https://aapm.onlinelibrary.wiley.com/doi/pdf/10.1118/1.4957690, https://doi.org/10.1118/1.4957690.

17. M.-C. Vozenin, J. Hendry, C. Limoli. Biological benefits of ultra-high dose rate flash radiotherapy: Sleeping beauty awoken, *Clinical Oncology*, 31 (7), 2019, 407–415. https://doi.org/10.1016/j.clon.2019.04.001.

18. S. Field, D. Bewley. Effects of dose-rate on the radiation response of rat skin, *International Journal of Radiation Biology and Related Studies in Physics, Chemistry and Medicine,* 26 (3), 1974, 259–267. doi: 10.1080/09553007414551221.

19. J. Bourhis, P. Montay-Gruel, P. Goncalves Jorge, C. Bailat, B. Petit, J. Ollivier, W. Jeanneret-Sozzi, M. Ozsahin, F. Bochud, R. Moeckli, J.-F. Germond, M.-C. Vozenin. Clinical translation of flash radiotherapy: Why and how? *Radiotherapy and Oncology*, 139, 2019, 11–17, FLASH radiotherapy International Workshop. https://doi.org/10.1016/j.radonc.2019.04.008. URL: https://www.sciencedirect.com/science/article/pii/S0167814019303603

20. M. Marinelli, G. Felici, F. Galante, A. Gasparini, L. Giuliano, S. Heinrich, M. Pacitti, G. Prestopino, V. Vanreusel, D. Verellen, C. Verona, G. Verona Rinati. Design, realization, and characterization of a novel diamond detector prototype for flash radiotherapy dosimetry, *Medical Physics*, 49 (3), 2022, 1902–1910. arXiv: https://aapm.onlinelibrary.wiley.com/doi/pdf/10.1002/mp.15473, https://doi.org/10.1002/mp.15473, URL: https://aapm.onlinelibrary.wiley.com/doi/abs/10.1002/mp.15473

21. M. Bazalova-Carter, B. Qu, B. Palma, B. H°ardemark, E. Hynning, C. Jensen, P. G. Maxim, B. W. Loo Jr. Treatment planning for radiotherapy with very high-energy electron beams and comparison of VHEE and VMAT plans, *Medical Physics*, 42 (5), 2015, 2615–2625. arXiv: https://aapm.onlinelibrary.wiley.com/doi/pdf/10.1118/1.4918923, https://doi.org/10.1118/1.4918923.

22. E. Schüler, K. Eriksson, E. Hynning, S. L. Hancock, S. M. Hiniker, M. Bazalova-Carter, T. Wong, Q.-T. Le, B. W. Loo Jr., P. G. Maxim. Very high-energy electron (VHEE) beams in radiation therapy: Treatment plan comparison between VHEE, VMAT, and PPBS, *Medical Physics*, 44 (6), 2017, 2544–2555. arXiv: https://aapm.onlinelibrary.wiley.com/doi/pdf/10.1002/mp.12233, doi: https://doi.org/10.1002/mp.12233.
23. D. S. M., et al. A data-driven fragmentation model for carbon therapy GPU-accelerated Monte-Carlo dose recalculation, *Frontiers in Oncology*, 12, 2022. doi: 10.3389/fonc.2022.780784.
24. A. Schiavi, et al. Fred: a GPU-accelerated fast-Monte Carlo code for rapid treatment plan recalculation in ion beam therapy, *Physics in Medicine and Biology*, 62 (18), 2017, 7482–7504. doi: 10.1088/1361-6560/aa8134.
25. G. Franciosini, G. Battistoni, A. Cerqua, A. D. Gregorio, P. D. Maria, M. D. Simoni, Y. Dong, M. Fischetti, M. Marafini, R. Mirabelli, A. Muscato, V. Patera, F. Salvati, A. Sarti, A. Sciubba, M. Toppi, G. Traini, A. Trigilio, A. Schiavi. GPU-accelerated Monte Carlo simulation of electron and photon interactions for radiotherapy applications, *Physics in Medicine & Biology*, 68 (4), 2023, 044001. doi: 10.1088/1361-6560/aca1f2.
26. A. Ferrari, et al. FLUKA: A multi-particle transport code (Program version 2005), CERN-2005-010, SLAC-R-773, INFN-TC-05-11, 2005.
27. H. Jiang, et al. Adaption of GEANT4 to Monte Carlo dose calculations based on CT data, *Med Phys*, 45, 2004, 459. doi: https://10.1118/1.1796952.
28. T. T. Bohlen, et al. Normal tissue sparing by flash as a function of single-fraction dose: A quantitative analysis, *International Journal of Radiation Oncology Biology Physics,* 2022. https://doi.org/10.1016/j.ijrobp.2022.05.038.
29. A. Sarti, et al. Deep seated tumour treatments with electrons of high energy delivered at flash rates: The example of prostate cancer, *Frontiers in Oncology,* 11, 2021, 5209. doi: 10.3389/fonc.2021.777852.
30. A. Muscato, L. Arsini, G. Battistoni, L. Campana, D. Carlotti, F. De Felice, A. De Gregorio, M. De Simoni, C. Di Felice, Y. Dong, G. Franciosini, M. Marafini, I. Mattei, R. Mirabelli, S. Muraro, M. Pacilio, L. Palumbo, V. Patera, A. Schiavi, A. Sciubba, M. Schwarz, S. Sorbino, V. Tombolini, M. Toppi, G. Traini, A. Trigilio, A. Sarti. Treatment planning of intracranial lesions with VHEE: comparing conventional and flash irradiation potential with state-of-the-art photon and proton radiotherapy, *Frontiers in Physics,* 11, 2023. doi: 10.3389/fphy.2023.1185598.

31. V. Favaudon, et al. Carboxyl radical induced cleavage of disulfide bonds in proteins: A gamma-ray and pulse radiolysis mechanistic investigation, *Biochemistry*, 29, 1990, 10978–10989.

32. L. Faillace, S. Barone, G. Battistoni, M. Di Francesco, G. Felici, L. Ficcadenti, G. Franciosini, F. Galante, L. Giuliano, L. Grasso, A. Mostacci, S. Muraro, M. Pacitti, L. Palumbo, V. Patera, M. Migliorati. Compact S-band linear accelerator system for ultrafast, ultrahigh dose-rate radiotherapy, *Phys. Rev. Accel. Beams*, 24, 2021, 050102. doi: 10.1103/PhysRevAccelBeams.24.050102., URL: https://link.aps.org/doi/10.1103/PhysRevAccelBeams.24.050102

33. M. El-Ashmawy, et al. Overall quality comparison of C-band and X-band medical linacs, in: Proceedings of the 14th Symposium on Accelerator Science and Technology, *The 14th Symposium on Accelerator Science and Technology*, Tsukuba, Japan, 2003, pp. 1–3.

34. T. Higo, et al. Advances in X-band TW accelerator structure operating in the 100 mv/m regime, in: Proceedings of IPAC'10, Kyoto, Japan, 2010, pp. 3702–3704.

35. E. I. Simakov, V. A. Dolgashev, S. G. Tantawi. Advances in high gradient normal conducting accelerator structures, *Nuclear Instruments and Methods in Physics Research Section A: Accelerators, Spectrometers, Detectors and Associated Equipment*, 907, 2018, 221–230 [advances in Instrumentation and Experimental Methods (Special Issue in Honour of Kai Siegbahn)]. https://doi.org/10.1016/j.nima.2018.02.085

36. V.A.Dolgashev,L.Faillace,B.Spataro,S.Tantawi,R.Bonifazi.High-gradient RF tests of welded X-band accelerating cavities, *Phys. Rev. Accel. Beams*, 24, 2021, 081002. doi: 10.1103/PhysRevAccelBeams.24.081002, URL: https://link.aps.org/doi/10.1103/PhysRevAccelBeams.24.081002

37. T. Sakurai, H. Ego, T. Inagaki, T. Asaka, D. Suzuki, S. Miura, Y. Otake. C-band disk-loaded-type accelerating structure for a high acceleration gradient and high-repetition-rate operation, *Phys. Rev. Accel. Beams*, 20, 2017, 042003. doi: 10.1103/PhysRevAccelBeams.20.042003, URL: https://link.aps.org/doi/10.1103/PhysRevAccelBeams.20.042003

38. W. Fang, Q. Gu, Z. Zhao, D. Tong. The C-band traveling-wave accelerating structure for compact XFEL at SINAP, in: Proceedings of IPAC2011, San Sebastián, Spain, 2011, pp. 133–135.

39. D. Alesini, M. Bellaveglia, M. Biagini, R. a Boni, M. Brönnimann, F. Cardelli, P. Chimenti, R. Clementi, G. Di Pirro, R. Di Raddo, M. Ferrario, L. Ficcadenti, A. Gallo, R. Kalt, V. Lollo, L. Palumbo, L. Piersanti, T. Schilcher. Design, realization and test of C-band accelerating structures for the

SPARC LAB linac energy upgrade, *Nuclear Instruments and Methods in Physics Research*, A 837, 2016, 161–170. http://dx.doi.org/10.1016/j.nima.2016.09.010.

40. D. Alesini, M. Bellaveglia, A. Bini S., Gallo, V. Lollo, L. Pellegrino, L. Piersanti, F. Cardelli, M. Migliorati, A. Mostacci, L. Palumbo, S. Tocci, L. Ficcadenti, V. Pettinacci. Design of high gradient, high repetition rate damped C-band RF structures, *Physical Review Accelerators and Beams,* 20, 2017. https://doi.org/10.1103/PhysRevAccelBeams.20.032004.

Chapter 5

Radiation Adaptive Response Effect: The History, Experiments, and Theoretical Models

Krzysztof Wojciech Fornalski
Faculty of Physics, Warsaw University of Technology, Poland
krzysztof.fornalski@pw.edu.pl

The traditional ionizing radiation dose-response approach has undergone a paradigm shift in recent decades, with many researchers challenging non-targeted effects through the exploration of the radiation adaptive response. This phenomenon, characterized by the protective response of cells or organisms to low doses or low-dose rates of ionizing radiation, has garnered significant attention due to its potential implications for radiation protection, cancer induction studies, and therapeutic interventions. Experimental activity in this field started more than 80 years ago, which is an interesting history of scientific investigations and people who uncovered more and more knowledge in this field. During the last two decades, a number of mathematical and biophysical models have played a crucial role in advancing the understanding of the radiation adaptive response.

Radioactivity in Life Sciences
Edited by Maria Letizia Terranova

ISBN 978-981-5129-67-0 (Hardcover), 978-1-003-63654-0 (eBook)
www.jennystanford.com

5.1 Introduction

The radiation adaptive response (or radioadaptation) is a radiobiological and biophysical phenomenon in which exposure to a low dose or dose rate of ionizing radiation primes cells or organisms to exhibit an enhanced resistance or repair capacity when subsequently exposed to higher, potentially damaging doses of radiation. This adaptive behavior challenges the traditional approach to radiation risk, which assumes a linear relationship between radiation dose and biological effects, even at low doses. The radiation adaptive response suggests that the relationship between dose and response is much more complex, particularly at lower levels of radiation exposure. One has to note, however, that this effect occurs relatively rarely, is difficult to predict, and the numerous cases of its occurrence observed are difficult to repeat. The radioadaptation is therefore an extremely complex effect that requires further detailed scientific research.

The radiation adaptive response effect can be observed in various experimental cases. The most frequent special case of radioadaptation is a priming dose effect, called Yonezawa or Raper-Yonezawa effect. The key characteristics of the Raper-Yonezawa effect include a priming dose, which is the initial exposure to low-level radiation, and a protective effect observed when cells or organisms encounter a challenging higher dose after the priming. The phenomenon exhibits dose dependence, with the magnitude of the adaptive response varying with the dose of the priming radiation. The temporal aspects are crucial, as the adaptive response is most effective when the challenging dose occurs after a specific time interval following the priming dose. Additionally, there is cell type specificity, meaning that different cell types and organisms may respond differently to the adaptive effects.

Another special case of the adaptive response is a constant low dose-rate irradiation. This can be found in high background radiation areas (HBRAa) studies, where inhabitants have been living for generations. The radioadaptation is observed for some of them as well.

Several proposed mechanisms attempt to explain the radiation adaptive response at the molecular and cellular levels. One hypothesis is that exposure to the priming dose or low dose rate stimulates cells to enhance their DNA repair mechanisms leading to more effective repair of radiation-induced damage during subsequent exposure. Another mechanism involves cell cycle regulation, where the priming dose induces changes in the cell cycle, causing a temporary arrest that allows for better repair before cell division. The activation of specific signaling pathways and changes in gene expression are also considered integral to the adaptive response, contributing to increased cell survival and protection against radiation-induced damage.

The implications of the radiation adaptive response are far-reaching. In radiation protection, if low doses induce protective responses, it challenges the assumptions of the linear no-threshold (LNT) model and may potentially influence the assessment of health risks associated with low-dose exposures. In radiation therapy, understanding the adaptive response has implications for treatment strategies, as it may be possible to exploit the adaptive response to selectively protect normal tissues while maintaining the therapeutic efficacy against cancer cells. On the other hand, the potential radioadaptation of cancerous cells can be very dangerous for patients.

However, the existence and relevance of the radiation adaptive response remain subjects of ongoing research and debate. While there is substantial experimental evidence supporting its occurrence, challenges and controversies persist, and researchers continue to explore the intricacies of this fascinating biological response to ionizing radiation. It is understandable that since we still do not know what exactly causes this effect, it should continue to be thoroughly investigated scientifically.

5.2 History of the Radiation Adaptive Response Studies

The first experimental studies on damage to chromosomes and their repairs were conducted in the 1930s by many radiobiologists, especially Karl Sax. In his 1939 paper entitled "The time factor in X-ray production of chromosome aberrations" [1], he found that negative effects are strictly related both to time and dose: "At low concentrations of irradiation these effects appear to be temporary and the cell recovers."

The next milestone was reached by John Raper who was a member of the Manhattan Project and conducted radiation research on mice, rats, and rabbits [2]. He irradiated animals with two consecutive doses: sublethal and much higher lethal. He obtained, for the first time, a specific hunchbacked curve of the adaptive response related to the time between both doses (Fig. 5.1). However, he could not fully explain what he observed because at that time DNA repair mechanisms were still not understood. John Raper called this effect "recovery from radiation damage." Raper's findings were confirmed a few years later by Eugene Cronkite and Collaborators [3] who stated that "it is concluded that no adequate explanation for this phenomenon of increased tolerance to X-ray radiation is available at present."

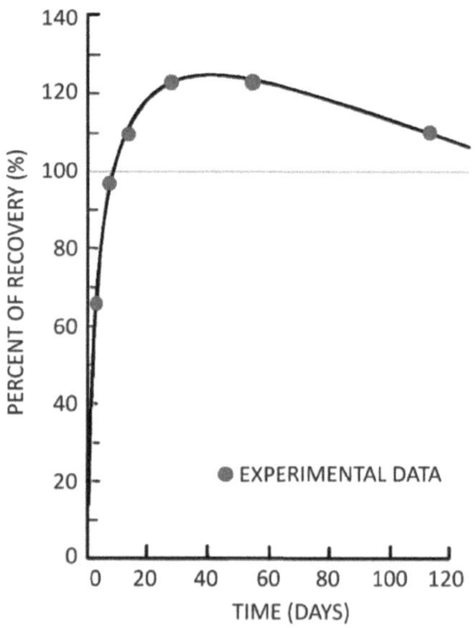

Figure 5.1 Results of animal experiments conducted by Dr John Raper during the Manhattan Project. The figure presents the percent of recovery of mice irradiated by beta radiation delivered in two doses (smaller sublethal and higher lethal). The horizontal axis represents the time between both doses (figure prepared based on data from J.R. Raper, "Effects of total surface beta irradiation," US Atomic Energy Commission, 1946 [2]).

Next experiments were conducted by Shields Warren and Arthur W. James who confirmed (in some single studies) that pre-exposure to X-rays could induce resistance to subsequent irradiation in mice.

Also, Elkind-Sutton experiments [4] were focused on the problem of cell recovery after irradiation of different doses and different radiation types.

After that, the studies on the radioadaptation were frozen because of a lack of new ideas and probably some political influences to show only the harmful effects of radioactivity. This situation lasted for almost two decades when J. Pohl-Rüling and P. Fisher concluded in 1979 that "these findings imply that protective mechanisms within the organism are capable of controlling the degree of radiation damage up to a certain point beyond which the effect again becomes dose-dependent" [5]. Finally, they found that "the shape of the dose-response curve at very low levels of radiation may result from the induction of repair enzymes." This was the next milestone: low radiation can enhance the production of repair enzymes.

The beginning of 1980 was a huge outpouring of scientific publications on this subject. Some of the lead scientists at that time were Gregorio Olivieri, Sheldon Wolff, Jeffrey Shadley, Andrzej Wójcik, Ron Mitchel, Edouard Azzam, Douglas Boreham, and G.Q. Dai [6–8]. In 1984, in the article "Adaptive response of human lymphocytes to low concentrations of radioactive thymidine" (*Science*, no. 223), the term "adaptive response" was used for the first time by G. Olivieri and Collaborators [9]. At the same time, advanced experimental investigations were conducted in Japan by Morio Yonezawa who irradiated mice with two consecutive doses: a small priming one and a second challenging one [10]. Based on his findings and experimental scheme, this special case of adaptive response was called the Yonezawa (or Raper-Yonezawa) effect [11], which is known as the priming dose effect in the US and Europe (Fig. 5.2 and Fig. 5.3). Parallelly, the radiation adaptive response was postulated to be a reason for the concept of radiation hormesis, which was popularized by Don Luckey.

The first overview of the radiation adaptive response effect (based mostly on the Yonezawa experimental scheme) was published by UNSCEAR in its 1994 report entitled "Adaptive responses to radiation in cells and organisms" [12] (UNSCEAR published the follow-up information in its 2020/2021 report, in Section III.F.4 [13]). At the same time, the second special case of adaptive response, namely low dose-rate irradiation in HBRAs was investigated, mostly in China and Iran (research was led by Javad Mortazavi).

At the beginning of the 21st century, the frequency of radioadaptation research decreased for the second time. However, during the last few years, new scientific studies appeared where different new irradiation schemes were tested, especially to discuss the adaptive response together with radiosensitivity [14].

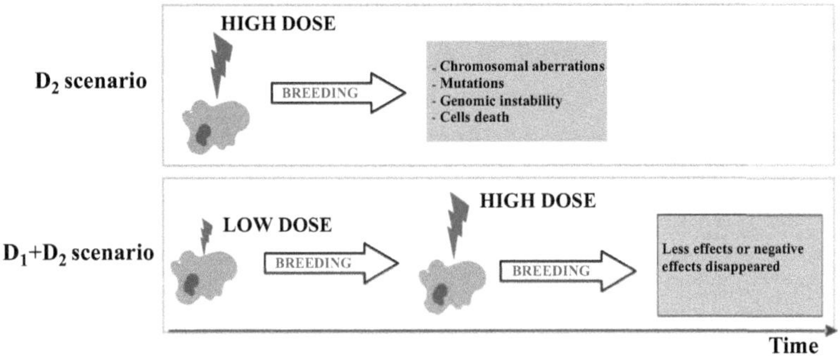

Figure 5.2 The simplified scheme of the priming dose effect (also called the Raper-Yonezawa effect), where the low priming dose is denoted as D_1, while the high challenging dose is D_2. The figure is based on the presentation of Prof. Marek Janiak (WIHE), 2008 (with permission).

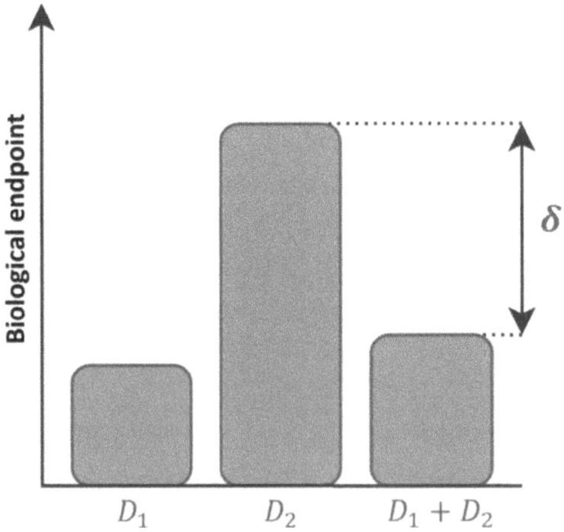

Figure 5.3 Schematical representation of the priming dose (Raper-Yonezawa) effect (see Fig. 5.2), the special case of the radiation adaptive response phenomenon. The difference between the group irradiated by the high challenging dose (D_2) and the group irradiated by two doses (priming and challenging, $D_1 + D_2$) is denoted as parameter δ (see Eq. (5.7)).

5.3 Mechanisms of the Radiation Adaptive Response

The radiation adaptive response is characterized by the ability of cells or organisms to exhibit increased resistance or repair mechanisms when exposed to low doses or low-dose rates of radiation before a subsequent higher radiation hazard [15, 16]. This in contrast to the conventional LNT model assumes a linear relationship between radiation dose and biological effects.

One of the primary mechanisms proposed for the radiation adaptive response involves the enhancement of DNA repair processes. Cells exposed to low doses of radiation may upregulate DNA repair pathways, allowing them to more efficiently repair DNA damage caused by subsequent higher doses.

Another mechanism is the induction of cell cycle arrest. Pre-exposure to low doses of radiation might lead to a temporary halt in the cell cycle, enabling cells to repair DNA damage before proceeding with cell division. This temporary pause could prevent the propagation of damaged DNA to daughter cells.

Radiation-induced oxidative stress is a known consequence of exposure to ionizing radiation. Low doses of radiation may stimulate the cell's antioxidant defenses, reducing overall oxidative damage caused by subsequent radiation exposure.

The activation of specific signaling pathways and changes in gene expression may play a crucial role in mediating the radiation adaptive response as well. Cells exposed to low doses of radiation may undergo changes in gene expression that promote cell survival and protect against subsequent radiation-induced damage.

In 2019, Yann Guéguen and Collaborators published a paper entitled "Adaptive responses to low doses of radiation or chemicals: their cellular and molecular mechanisms" [17], which discussed the similarities between radiation and other agents that trigger adaptation of the organism. They reviewed the recent knowledge of radioadaptation, which is based on the following complex effects:

- improved detoxification of free radicals,
- enhancement of DNA repair systems,
- induction of new proteins,
- enhanced antioxidant production,

- enhanced immune/inflammatory response,
- cell cycle regulation, and
- induction of apoptosis.

Nevertheless, many mechanisms of the radiation adaptive response are known, however, we still do not know the most important aspect: what is the trigger for the effect appearance? This still needs further scientific investigation because radioadaptation is very complex and still not fully understood [18].

5.4 Problems and Main Issues with the Radioadaptation

While the radiation adaptive response is a fascinating phenomenon with potential implications for radiation protection and therapy, there are several challenges, controversies, and areas of uncertainty associated with this concept. Here are some of the problems and limitations associated with the radiation adaptive response:

- **Inconsistent replication of effects:** One significant challenge is the inconsistency in replicating the radiation adaptive response across different studies and experimental setups. Some studies fail to observe the protective effects associated with low-dose priming, leading to questions about the robustness and reliability of the phenomenon.
- **Cell type specificity:** The adaptive response may vary among different cell types, tissues, and organisms. The mechanisms and effectiveness of the response can differ, making it challenging to generalize findings across diverse biological systems. Understanding the factors that contribute to this cell type specificity is an ongoing area of research.
- **Dose and temporal dependence:** The radiation adaptive response is dose-dependent, and its effectiveness may vary with the dose of the priming radiation. Additionally, for the Raper-Yonezawa scheme, the timing between the priming dose and the challenging dose is crucial as well. The dose and temporal dependencies complicate the application of the adaptive response concept in practical scenarios.

- **Relevance to human health:** While laboratory studies have provided valuable insights, translating the findings to the complex interplay of factors influencing human health is challenging. Epidemiological studies attempting to link the adaptive response to lower cancer rates in certain populations living in areas with higher background radiation levels have yielded mixed results, and the overall relevance to human health remains uncertain.
- **Complexity of mechanisms:** The precise molecular mechanisms underlying the radiation adaptive response are not fully understood. Multiple potential mechanisms have been proposed, including DNA repair enhancement, cell cycle regulation, and activation of signaling pathways, as described in previous chapters. The complexity of these mechanisms presents challenges in unraveling the specific pathways involved [18].
- **Controversies in radiation protection:** The existence of the radiation adaptive response challenges the assumptions of the linear no-threshold (LNT) model, which forms the basis for radiation protection standards. Controversies arise regarding how to integrate the adaptive response into radiation protection guidelines, as it may influence the assessment of health risks associated with low-dose exposures. However, it is still difficult to precisely determine the exact influence of the adaptive response to the general human radiation risk.
- **Risk-benefit considerations in radiation therapy:** In the context of radiation therapy, the radiation adaptive response introduces complexities in determining the optimal balance between therapeutic efficacy and potential protective effects on normal tissues. Understanding how to exploit the adaptive response to enhance treatment outcomes without compromising cancer cell killing remains a challenge. An additional issue is connected with the potential radioadaptation of cancer cells, where the effect is negative (potential enhancement of cancer cells' survival rate).
- **Bystander effect and other non-targeted responses:** The role of bystander effects, where non-irradiated cells exhibit responses similar to irradiated cells, adds another layer of

complexity. The interplay between targeted and non-targeted responses in the adaptive process is not fully elucidated, and the implications for therapeutic strategies and radiation protection are not yet well-defined. Generally, both the radioadaptive and negative results are observed among bystander cells.

5.5 Modeling of the Radiation Adaptive Response

During the last two decades several theoretical propositions of the adaptive response description were published because, so far, there are a lot of experimental findings without a broader and general view. More than that, large deviations of experimental data, huge statistical fluctuations, and different cells and organisms used for investigations, make it difficult to find answers to the most important questions and to generalize the description of the adaptive response effect.

The first model that mathematically describes the effect of the radiation adaptive response in a priming dose scheme is the multi-parameter, phenomenological model of Morio Yonezawa and Olga Smirnova, which was published in two consecutive papers in the Health Physics journal in 2003 and 2004 [19, 20]. The model describes the impact of ionizing radiation on hematopoiesis, a system critical to the proper functioning of the body. Hematopoiesis consists of four main processes, each of which is responsible for the formation of different blood cells: thrombopoiesis, which is responsible for the formation of thrombocytes; erythropoiesis, which is responsible for the formation of erythrocytes; lymphopoiesis, which is responsible for the formation of lymphocytes; and granulopoiesis, which is responsible for the formation of granulocytes. Each of the mentioned processes contains a set of cells, from bone marrow stem cells, which predefine the type of a given cell, to mature cells that make up the blood. Generally, the authors' model proposed a deterministic description of the impact of ionizing radiation on cells of those four main blood cell lines (thrombocytes, lymphocytes, erythrocytes, and granulocytes). The model assumes the division of cells into categories according to the stage of their development (bone marrow stem cells, maturing and undivided precursor cells, and mature blood cells) and according to the damage suffered (undamaged cells, damaged cells, and severely damaged cells), and it describes the relationships between these categories. The model uses systems of many differential equations (different numbers of equations for subsequent blood cell lines) containing many free parameters that must be determined based on experimental data. The proposed model allows for the simulation of both radiation pulses (including irradiation in the Raper-Yonezawa scheme) as well as chronic irradiation with a certain dose rate (Fig. 5.4). It should be noted that the limitations of applying to only a few cell types, as well as the large number of free parameters, significantly reduce the practical usefulness of the model.

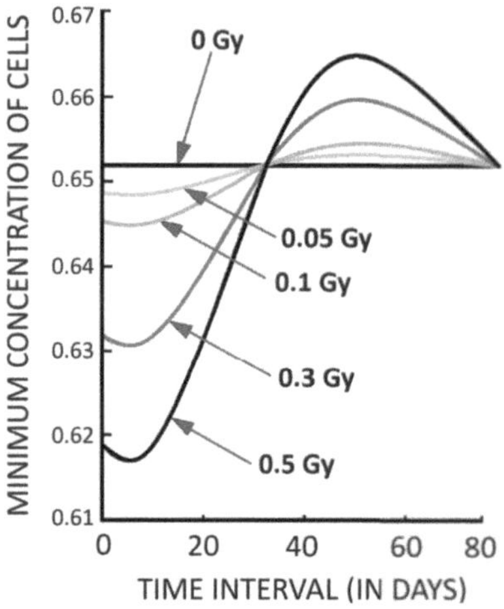

Figure 5.4 Example of Yonezawa & Smirnova model application: minimal concentrations of granulocytes after acute irradiation at dose D = 4 Gy vs. the duration of the time interval between this challenge exposure and preliminary priming dose irradiation with doses presented with arrows. The figure was created based on the data of Ref. [19] (with permission).

Another interesting model, which describes the radiation adaptive response in the priming dose (Raper-Yonezawa) scheme, is the Italian model authored by Giuseppe Esposito and Collaborators in 2011 [21]. This model was developed based on the Lethal-Potentially Lethal (LPL) model (popular in radiation biophysics) describing cellular survival curves. The Italian model determines the level of protective effect of the priming dose depending on the time that has passed since absorbing a small dose, also taking into account both the dose value and the dose-rate value (Fig. 5.5). The model introduced a number of variables, defined by a system of differential equations, describing, among others: the rate of cell repair, the level of free radicals generated by ionizing radiation, and the level of antioxidant enzymes. In order to explain the occurrence of the radiation adaptive response, the authors focused on the increased efficiency of DNA repair and the production of antioxidant enzymes as a result of irradiation with the priming dose. According to the original LPL model, damaged cells were divided into two categories: cells whose damage is potentially lethal and cells whose damage is definitely lethal. Potentially lethal damage can be properly repaired by the body's repair mechanisms, including antioxidant enzymes. This type of damage can also be repaired incorrectly, in which case such damage becomes lethal. The authors used the number of lethally damaged cells as a determinant of the adaptive response. It was assumed that the adaptive response is characterized by a lower number of lethal lesions compared to the number of lethal lesions when the adaptive response did not occur [21].

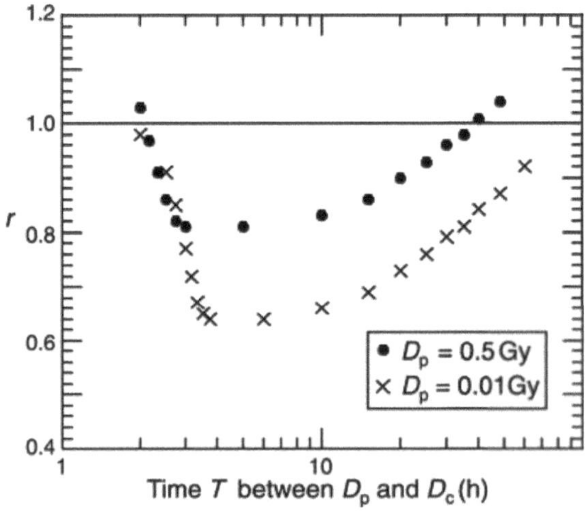

Figure 5.5 The adaptive response factor, r, in the function of time between priming (D_p) and challenging (D_c) doses in the Italian model. The figure is based on Ref. [21] (with permission).

Modeling of adaptive response and radiosensitivity is also conducted by Nicolas Foray and his team (Fig. 5.6). They published several papers describing different aspects of those phenomena [22–25]. One approach uses the linear-quadratic (LQ) model, popular in radiobiology, which is usually applied to describing the survival fraction of a cell colony. Thanks to this, Foray's model makes it possible to determine the occurrence and level of the radiation adaptive response by analyzing the number of double-strand DNA lesions and the number of Ataxia-Telangiectasia Mutated (ATM) monomers involved in DNA repair processes, depending on the radiation dose received and the time that has passed since its receipt [25]. The basic assumption of the model is the possibility of its interpretation from a biological perspective, and in particular explaining: (a) the impact of ionizing radiation in a wide range of doses, (b) the radiosensitivity of certain genes caused by mutations in cytoplasmic proteins, and (c) the phenomenon of hyper-radiosensitivity to low doses of radiation. The authors' model postulated that ionizing radiation leads to the oxidation of ATM dimers, which, in turn, trigger ATM monomerization with an intensity proportional to the radiation dose received. The resulting monomers diffuse into the cell nucleus and then enable the recognition of double-strand breaks of DNA through the phosphorylation of histones H2AX (γH2AX), ultimately repairing such damage. Among the unrepaired double-strand breaks, only some contribute to cell death (the remaining damage is tolerated by them). This hypothesis leads to a coherent biomathematical and molecular interpretation of the LQ model, considering recognized but unrepaired double-strand breaks and unrecognized double-strand breaks as cell lethal events [25].

Other models are also dedicated to the priming dose (Raper-Yonezawa) scheme and usually are not connected to a much broader and general approach to the adaptive response. However, let us mention that those models were created by prominent scientists like Bobby Leonard, Bobby Scott, Dominik Wodarz, Yehoshua Socol, Katsuhito Kino, and many others [26, 27].

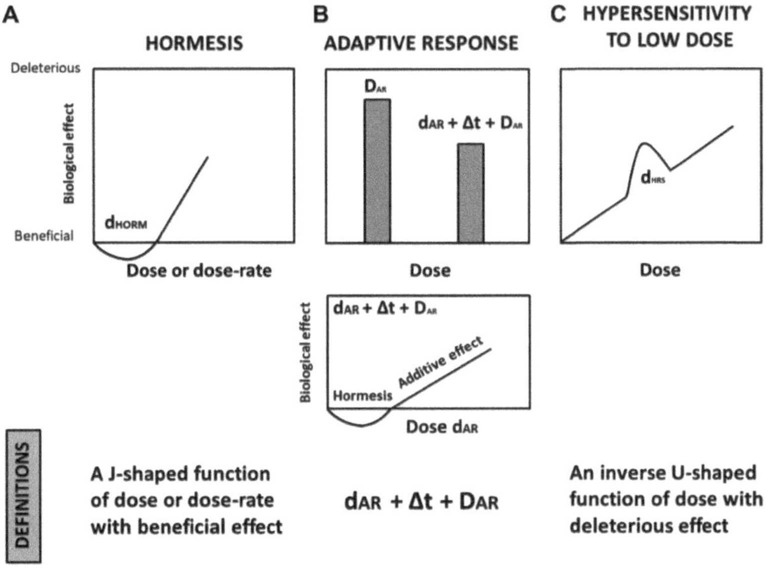

Figure 5.6 Main assumptions of the French adaptive response model, where authors applied the effect to the dose-response risk function with hormetic shape. The figure is based on Ref. [24] (with permission).

5.6 Dual Response Probability Model: Feinendegen's Approach

The very interesting model of the adaptive response was formulated by Prof. Ludwig Feinendegen, a prominent figure in the field of radiation biology and radiation medicine. His scientific work has focused on elucidating the mechanisms and implications of low-dose radiation effects, including the phenomenon of radiation hormesis and the adaptive response. Feinendegen's model of the radiation adaptive response is part of his broader research into the health effects of low-dose radiation [28–32].

Feinendegen's model of the radiation adaptive response incorporates the concept of radiation hormesis, which posits that low doses of a stressor (such as radiation) can have a beneficial effect, while higher doses may be harmful. Therefore, the adaptive response is applied by the model as the main basis for the hormetic response (Fig. 5.7). The key features of Feinendegen's model include:

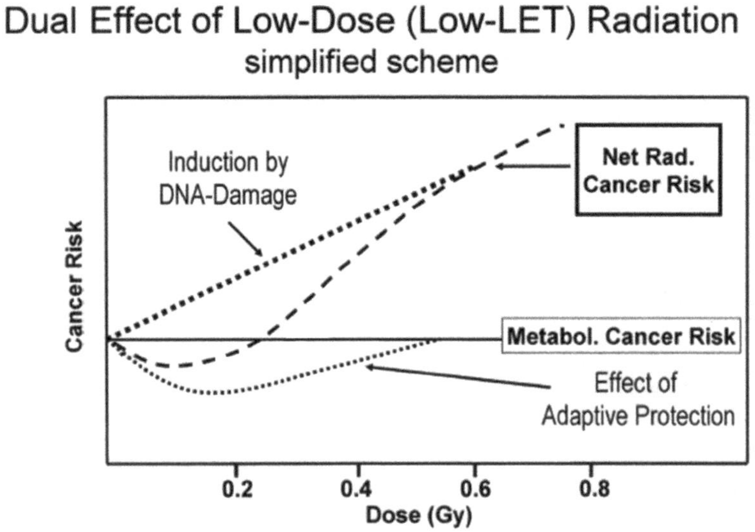

Figure 5.7 The main concept of the Feinendegen's model, where detrimental effects (DNA-Damage linear relationship) are balanced by the effect of adaptive protection. The figure is based on Ref. [30] (with permission).

- **Threshold-like behavior:** Feinendegen's model suggests that there is a threshold-like behavior in the response to low-dose radiation. Below a certain dose, the radiation-induced effects may be beneficial or adaptive, activating protective mechanisms within cells and organisms. Above the threshold, the dose-response is simply linear (Fig. 5.7).
- **Biphasic response:** The model proposes a biphasic response to radiation, with low doses inducing an adaptive response that protects against subsequent damage. This is called the hormetic region. Higher doses, however, may overwhelm the adaptive capacity, leading to a more traditional linear or sublinear response.
- **Biological defense mechanisms:** Feinendegen emphasizes the role of biological defense mechanisms activated by low doses of radiation. These mechanisms may include enhanced DNA repair, apoptosis (programmed cell death) of damaged cells, and other cellular processes that contribute to maintaining genomic stability. This is generally consistent with the recent knowledge about the effect, which was mentioned in previous chapters.

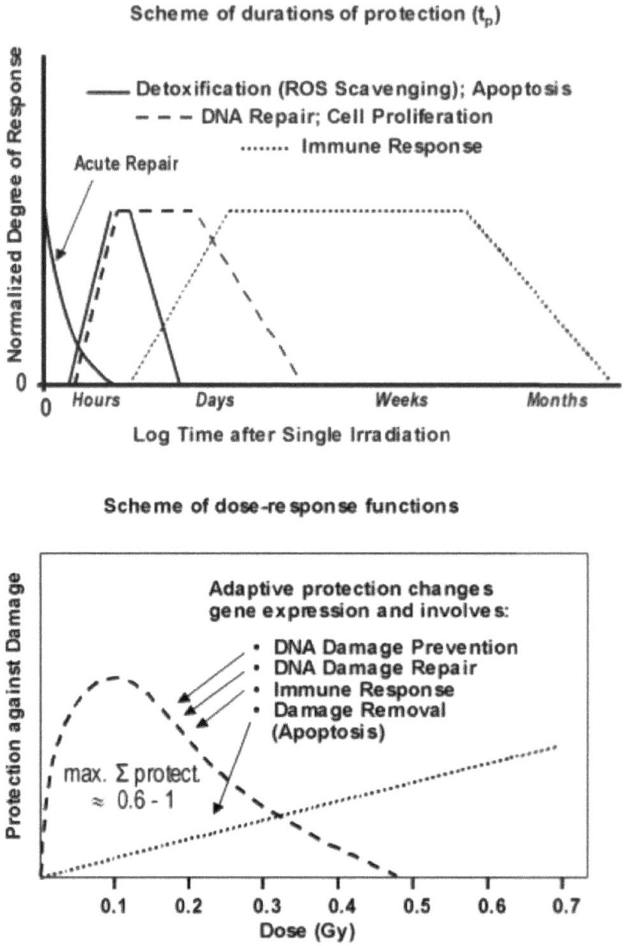

Figure 5.8 Two functions of the radiation adaptive response in the Feinendegen's model: the time-related function of repair (top plot) and the dose-related hunchbacked function (bottom plot). The figure is based on Ref. [30] (with permission).

- **Stress response pathways:** The model incorporates stress response pathways, which are activated in response to low-dose radiation. These pathways may involve various signaling molecules and gene expression changes, leading to an overall enhancement of cellular resilience.

- **Experimental evidence and support:** The model is supported by experimental evidence from both in vitro and in vivo studies. For example, Feinendegen's research has shown that pre-exposure to low doses of radiation can induce an adaptive response, reducing the genomic instability and mutagenic effects observed after subsequent higher doses in the Raper-Yonezawa scheme. However, the model is based on data from other scientific groups as well.
- **Dose and time aspects:** The crucial relationship for the model is a dose-response function which is a result of positive (hormetic) or negative factors (Fig. 5.7). Therefore, Feinendegen uses the hunchbacked curve to describe the adaptive response curve dependent on the dose (Fig. 5.8). Additionally, the time factor is implemented, and the time-related actions are results of previous dose activity. This creates two adaptive relationships: dose and time-dependent (Fig. 5.8), which are joined into one function called $p_{AR}(D, t)$.

Feinendegen defined the cancer risk (R), which is equivalent to the radiation risk probability function for a person irradiated by ionizing radiation (D):

$$R = P_{ind}D - p_{AR}(D,t) \cdot (R_{spo} + P_{ind}D) \quad (5.1)$$

where $P_{ind}\,D$ is an LNT term (radiation-induced lethal cancer risk), p_{AR} is dose- and time-related probability function of the adaptive response, and R_{spo} is a spontaneous lifetime cancer risk of the exposed individual.

Feinendegen calculated all parameters' values on experimental data to assess the cancer risk under those assumptions. A few years later he proposed a simplified version of Eq. (5.1):

$$R = P_{ind}D - p_{AR}R_{spo} \quad (5.2)$$

which has, in fact, the same result: the overall cancer risk is a balancing process between beneficial and detrimental factors. This philosophy was enhanced by Fornalski [33, 34], where no single but many beneficial and detrimental factors are dancing around the balance (equilibrium) state, what biologists call homeostasis (Fig. 5.9).

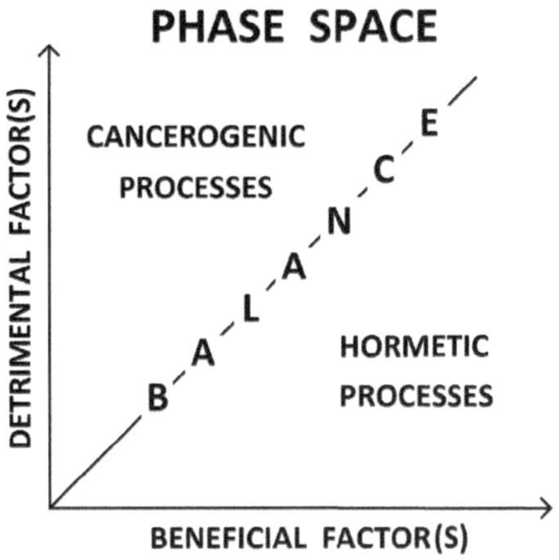

Figure 5.9 The generalization of the Feinendegen approach made by K. Fornalski, where various negative (cancerogenic) and positive (hormetic) processes are balanced around the equilibrium state (homeostasis). The figure is based on Ref. [33] (with permission).

5.7 Three-Parameter Biophysical Model

The recent phenomenological and fully biophysical model was proposed by Krzysztof Fornalski in 2014 [35] and developed during the next years in cooperation with Ludwik Dobrzyński and Collaborators [36, 37] in the National Centre for Nuclear Research (NCBJ), Poland. However, the most recent calculations and applications to experimental data were conducted by K. Fornalski and his students in the Physics of Complex Systems Division at the Faculty of Physics, Warsaw University of Technology, Poland [38].

The model is a stochastic one that is based on the probability of occurrence of an adaptive response caused by ionizing radiation. The model does not place any restrictions on the specific irradiation regimen in which it can be used. Therefore, it is possible to use it in the Raper-Yonezawa scheme, in the scheme of irradiation with multiple pulses of priming doses, or in the scheme of chronic irradiation with a certain dose rate [38]. The model can be used both in DNA damage analysis and DNA mutation analysis. The δ parameter was introduced in the model to objectively assess the level of the induced adaptive response (Fig. 5.3). The value taken by this parameter indicates how significant the damage/mutations produced by a given irradiation scheme compared to irradiation at the target (challenging) dose only.

The model places great emphasis on ease of use and universality. Thus, the introduced parameter δ depends only on three free parameters, which must be determined experimentally. There are also no restrictions on the type of cells to which the model can be applied. However, due to possible differences in the nature of the adaptive response depending on the cell type, in order to ensure the correct operation of the model, it must be calibrated (calibration involves experimental determination of α parameters) separately for each cell category.

The important thing is that the model is based on many approaches presented by Feinendegen, especially the hunchbacked shape of crucial curves. Therefore, the probability functions of the adaptive response appearance may be described as separate dose- and time-dependent hunchbacked equations [35]:

$$P(D) = \beta_1 D^2 \exp(-\alpha_1 D) \tag{5.3}$$

$$P(t) = \beta_2 t^2 \exp(-\alpha_2 t) \tag{5.4}$$

where D is a radiation dose received t time ago, while $\alpha_{1,2}$ and $\beta_{1,2}$ are free parameters. Those two equations may be combined into a single joint formula that describes the final probability function of radiation adaptive response appearance [35]:

$$p_{AR}(D,t) = \alpha_0 D^2 t^2 \exp(-\alpha_1 D - \alpha_2 t) \tag{5.5}$$

Equation (5.5) is universal one and can be applied to many doses (dose pulses) as a simple sum of $P_{AR,total} = \Sigma p_{AR}$ (see Fig. 5.10). Analogically, this formula can be presented in continuous form, where the general dose-rate time distribution, $\dot{D}(t)$, with τ as a cell's (or organism's) age, can be applied, instead of dose pulses as previously. Therefore:

$$P_{AR,\text{total}} = \int_{t=0}^{\tau} p_{AR}\left(\dot{D}, \tau - t\right) dt \tag{5.6}$$

This is a basis for the model, which was presented originally in 2014 [35]. During the next years, the model was successfully applied to describe, e.g., the Raper-Yonezawa effect [37], as well as constant low dose-rate irradiation [36].

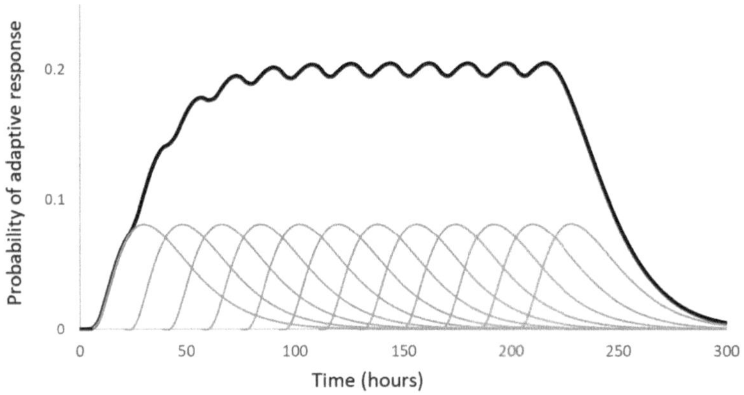

Figure 5.10 Exemplary application of the model proposed by K. Fornalski [38]: the black solid curve represents the total adaptive response function, $P_{AR,total}$, which is a sum of single hunchbacked curves given by Eq. (5.5) (in grey). Each grey curve is an adaptive response signal generated by a dose pulse delivered every 6 hours for model parameters calibrated for human lymphocytes in vitro: α_0 = 22.9 Gy^{-2}h^{-3}, α_1 = 79.4 Gy^{-1}, and α_2 = 0.0832 h^{-1}. This scheme of irradiation (dose pulses delivered with some time shift) is called "radiation training."

5.7.1 Special Case of the Raper-Yonezawa Effect [37]

In the special case of the Raper-Yonezawa effect, one can define the delta parameter as:

$$\delta = 1 - \frac{N_{1+2}}{N_2} \tag{5.7}$$

where N_2 corresponds to the number of DNA lesions or mutations in a single dose D_2 scenario, while N_{1+2} is the number of such biological endpoints in a D_1+D_2 case scenario (with time interval, Δt, between both doses) (see Fig. 5.2 and Fig. 5.3). The value of N can be simply denoted as $N = \mu\ D$, which is consistent with linear relationships of early physical damages in the cellular DNA. However, repair mechanisms, which are enhanced by adaptive response, can reduce the value of N as $dN = -\ N\ P_{AR,total}\ dt$, which is a crucial point of this approach. Please note that $P_{AR,total}$ for the time $T > \Delta t$ is composed of two functions given by Eq. (5.5), namely $P_{AR,total} = p_{AR}(D_1,T) + p_{AR}(D_2,T\text{-}\Delta t)$. Therefore the priming dose, D_1, strongly enhances the value of $P_{AR,total}$, which, in the next step, enhances the reduction of N.

5.7.2 Priming Dose Received in the Long Time Period [38]

The classical Raper-Yonezawa effect assumes that both doses, D_1 and D_2, are applied in a very short time each, as mentioned as "dose pulses." However, in many experimental cases, both doses can be delivered during quite long periods with a constant dose rate. When irradiation starts, the adaptive response function is summarized and only time-dependent (dose rate, $\dot{D}$, is constant):

$$P_{AR,total}(t) = \int_0^t p_{AR} dt = \xi_{\dot{D}} \left(1 - e^{-\alpha_2 t}\left[\frac{1}{2}(\alpha_2 t)^2 + \alpha_2 t + 1\right]\right) \quad (5.8)$$

where $\xi_{\dot{D}} = 2\alpha_0 \alpha_2^{-3} \dot{D}^2 \exp(-\alpha_1 \dot{D})$. The function given by Eq. (5.8) saturates to some constant value (see next subchapter), but when the irradiation stops after some time τ, the probability function of the adaptive response disappears as:

$$P_{AR,total}(T > \tau) = \xi_{\dot{D}} \int_0^{\tau} (T-t)^2 e^{-\alpha_2 (T-t)} dt$$

$$= \frac{1}{2}\xi_{\dot{D}} \begin{bmatrix} e^{\alpha_2(\tau - T)}\left(\alpha_2(T-\tau)\left[\alpha_2(T-\tau)+2\right]+2\right) \\ +e^{-\alpha_2 T}\left(-\alpha_2 T\left[\alpha_2 T + 2\right] - 2\right) \end{bmatrix} \quad (5.9)$$

which is valid only when the analyzed moment T is oriented after the irradiation time, τ. Thus, the probability function of the adaptive response given by Eq. (5.9) shall be used in the moment of D_2 appearance when τ is long enough (see the right-hand side of Fig. 5.10, where the black curve is decreasing).

5.7.3 Constant Low Dose-Rate Irradiation [36]

When the irradiation time is long enough, the function given by Eq. (5.8) saturates, and the constant probability of adaptive response equals:

$$P_{AR,total} \equiv P_C = \lim_{t \to \infty} \int_0^t p_{AR}(\dot{D}, t) dt = \alpha_3' \dot{D}^2 \exp(-\alpha_1' \dot{D}) \quad (5.10)$$

with new constants α_1' and α_3' because of changing the dose D into dose rate $\dot{D}$ (change of units). Equation (5.10) can be applied whenever such long-time saturation to constant P_C is expected, e.g., in high background radiation areas (HBRAs) or during long deep space travels (which can be called a Mortazavi scheme of radioadaptation). This is represented by the plateau in Fig. 5.10.

To conclude, the presented model developed by Fornalski and his Team [38] assumes that the adaptive response function (p_{AR}) is strictly related to the effectiveness of DNA lesions (N) repair. The higher the actual value of p_{AR}, the stronger the N decrease. This can determine the relative difference between adapted and control groups (δ), e.g., with high dose (HD) and low dose (LD). The great advantage of the model is that p_{AR} function can have different forms regarding radiation doses (or dose rates) distribution, e.g., single dose, two doses, multiple doses, or a constant dose rate. This makes the model very universal for every type of irradiation, but needs some mathematical calculations based on three basic model equations:

$$\begin{cases} p_{AR} = \alpha_0 D^2 t^2 \exp\left(-\alpha_1 D - \alpha_2 t\right) \\ dN = -N p_{AR} dt \\ \delta = 1 - N_{HD|LD} / N_{HD} \end{cases} \tag{5.11}$$

5.8 Conclusions

The radiation adaptive response stands as a captivating and complex phenomenon that challenges traditional models of radiation biology and biophysics. While the simple linear no-threshold model has long served as a practical approximation for the general dose-response function, the adaptive response suggests that the relationship between radiation dose and biological effects is more nuanced than previously thought.

Mathematical and biophysical models, such as those proposed by Ludwig Feinendegen or other authors (see Figs. 5.11, 5.12, and 5.13), provide valuable frameworks for understanding the radiation adaptive response. These models integrate the complexities of cellular responses, dose dependencies, and temporal dynamics, contributing to a more comprehensive understanding of the adaptive mechanisms at play. The last presented model was proposed by Fornalski, and—as opposed to other models—it contains only three parameters: α_0 responsible for probability function normalization, α_1 responsible for the optimal dose application, and α_2 for the time relationship. It seems that all those parameters vary due to the different types of cells, species, or tissues. Anyway, this needs to be investigated in the future regarding the individual radiosensitivity of different organisms.

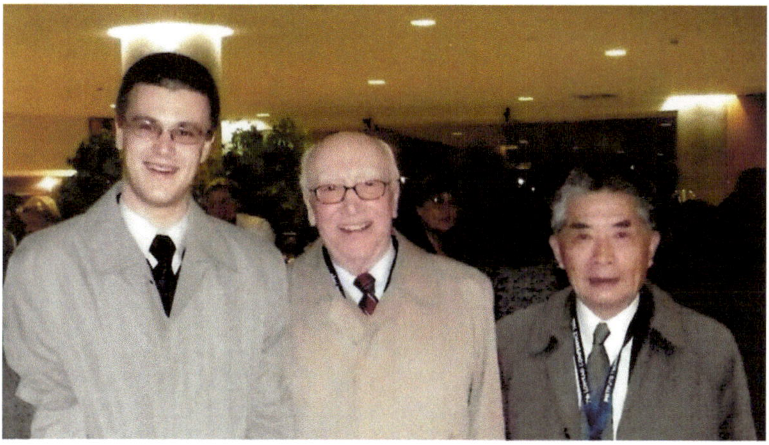

Figure 5.11 At the LOWRAD 2008 Conference in Lisbon, Portugal. From the left: K. Fornalski, L. Feinendegen, and H. Tanooka.

As technology and research methods continue to advance, the intricacies of the radiation adaptive response will likely become clearer. It is very important because radioadaptation is still not fully understood, and much experimental research failed to clearly demonstrate the effect. However, the ongoing dialogue between physicists, biologists, and clinicians is vital for translating scientific findings into practical applications that improve both the safety of radiation exposure and the effectiveness of radiation therapy in treating various medical conditions. The radiation adaptive response stands as a testament to the dynamic interplay between living organisms and their environment, challenging our preconceptions and opening new avenues for exploration in the field of radiation biology and radiation biophysics.

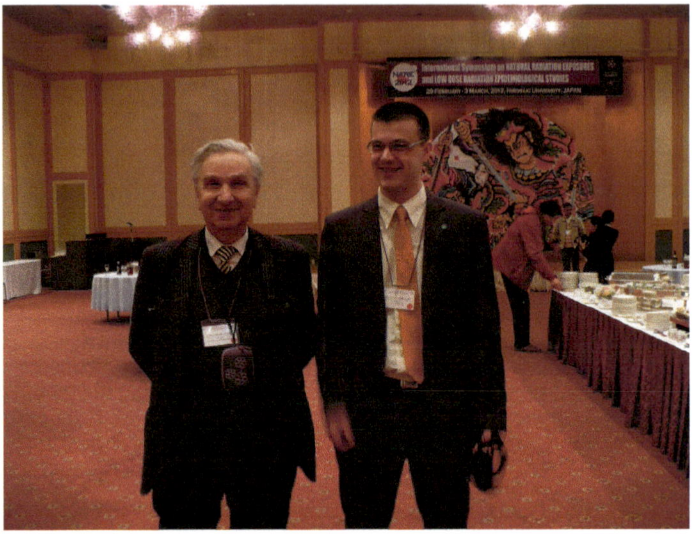

Figure 5.12 At the NARE 2012 Conference, Hirosaki, Japan. From the left: L. Dobrzyński and K. Fornalski.

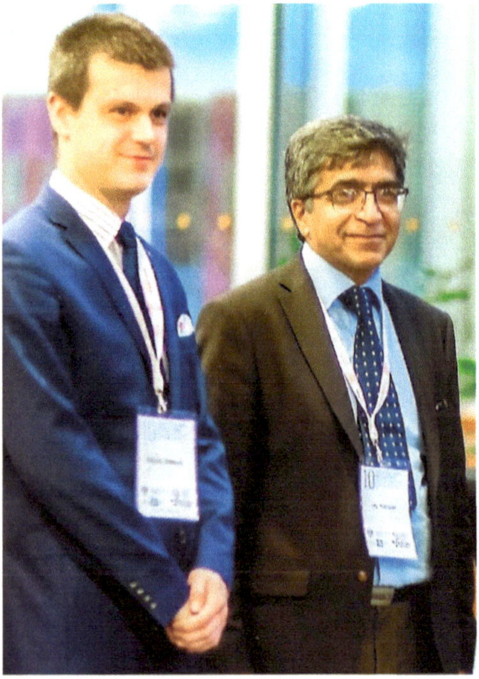

Figure 5.13 Tenth Nuclear Power Conference 2018 in Warsaw, Poland. From the left: K. Fornalski and J. Mortazavi.

References

1. Sax K. (1939) The time factor in X-ray production of chromosome aberrations. *Proceedings of the National Academy of Sciences*, 25(5), 225–233.
2. Raper J.R. (1947) Effects of total surface beta irradiation. *Radiology*, 49, 314–324.
3. Cronkite E.P., Sipe C.R., Eltzholtz D.C., Chapman W.H., Chambers F.W. (1950) Increased tolerance of mice to lethal X-radiation as a result of previous sublethal exposures. *Proc. Soc. Exp. Biol. Med.*, 73, 184–186.
4. Elkind M.M., Sutton H. (1959) X-ray damage and recovery in mammalian cells in culture. *Nature*, 184, 1293–1295.
5. Pohl-Rüling J., Fischer P. (1979) The dose-effect relationship of chromosome aberrations to alpha and gamma irradiation in a population subjected to an increased burden of natural radioactivity. *Radiation Research*, 80(1), 61–81.
6. Mitchel R.E.J. (2009) The dose window for radiation-induced protective adaptive responses. *Dose Response*, 8(2), 192–208.
7. Shadley J.D., Afzal V., Wolff S. (1987) Characterization of the adaptive response to ionizing radiation induced by low doses of X-rays to human lymphocytes. *Radiation Research*, 111(3), 511–517.
8. Wolff S. (1998) The adaptive response in radiobiology: evolving insights and implications. *Environmental Health Perspectives*, 106(1), 277–283.
9. Olivieri G., Bodycote J., Wolff S. (1984) Adaptive response of human lymphocytes to low concentrations of radioactive thymidine. *Science*, 223, 594–597.
10. Yonezawa M, Misonoh J, Hosokawa Y. (1990) Acquired radioresistance after small dose X-irradiation in mice. *J Radiat Res.*, 31(3), 256–262.
11. Wang B., Tanaka K., Ninomiya Y., Maruyama K., Vares G., Eguchi-Kasai K., Nenoi M. (2013) Relieved residual damage in the hematopoietic system of mice rescued by radiation-induced adaptive response (Yonezawa Effect). *J Radiat Res.*, 54(1), 45–51.
12. UNSCEAR (United Nations Scientific Committee on the Effects of Atomic Radiation) 1994 Report, "Sources and effects of ionizing radiation". Annex B: Adaptive responses to radiation in cells and organisms.
13. UNSCEAR (United Nations Scientific Committee on the Effects of Atomic Radiation) 2020/2021 Report Volume III, "Sources, effects and

risks of ionizing radiation". Annex C: Biological mechanisms relevant for the inference of cancer risks from low-dose and low-dose-rate radiation. Section III.F.4 "Adaptive response".

14. Fornalski K.W. (2019) Radiation adaptive response and cancer: from the statistical physics point of view. *Physical Review E*, 99(2), article no. 022139.
15. Tapio S., Jacob V. (2007) Radioadaptive response revisited. *Radiat Environ Biophys*, 46, 1–12.
16. Dimova E.G., Bryant P.E., Chankova S.G. (2008) Adaptive response: some underlying mechanisms and open questions. *Genet. Mol. Biol.*, 31(2).
17. Guéguen Y., Bontemps A., Ebrahimian T.G. (2019) Adaptive responses to low doses of radiation or chemicals: their cellular and molecular mechanisms. *Cellular and Molecular Life Sciences*, 76, 1255–1273.
18. Piotrowski Ł., Krasowska J., Fornalski K.W. (2023) Mechanistic modelling of DNA damage repair by the radiation adaptive response mechanism and its significance. *BioMedInformatics*, 3(1), 150–163.
19. Smirnova O.A., Yonezawa M. (2003) Radioprotection effect of low-level pre-irradiation on mammals: modeling and experimental investigations. *Health Physics*, 85(2), 150–158.
20. Smirnova O.A., Yonezawa M. (2004) Radioresistance in mammals induced by low-level chronic irradiation: modeling and experimental investigations. *Health Phys.*, 87(4), 366–374.
21. Esposito G., Campa A., Pinto M., Simone G., Tabocchini M.A., Belli M. (2010) Adaptive response: modelling and experimental studies. *Radiation Protection Dosimetry*, 143(2–4), 320–324.
22. Foray N., Charvet A.-M., Duchemin D., Favaudon V., Lavalette D. (2005) The repair rate of radiation-induced DNA damage: a stochastic interpretation based on the Gamma function. *Journal of Theoretical Biology*, 236(4), 448–458. doi: 10.1016/j.jtbi.2005.03.027
23. Devic C., Ferlazzo M.L., Foray N. (2018) Influence of individual radiosensitivity on the adaptive response phenomenon: toward a mechanistic explanation based on the nucleo-shuttling of ATM protein. *Dose-Response*, 16(3).
24. Devic C., Ferlazzo M.L., Berthel E., Foray N. (2020) Influence of individual radiosensitivity on the hormesis phenomenon: toward a mechanistic explanation based on the nucleo-shuttling of ATM protein. *Dose-Response*, 18(2).

25. Bodgi L., Foray N. (2016) The nucleo-shuttling of the atm protein as a basis for a novel theory of radiation response: resolution of the linear-quadratic model. *International Journal of Radiation Biology*, 92(3), 117–131.
26. Socol Y., Shaki Y., Dobrzyński L. (2020) Damped-oscillator model of adaptive response and its consequences. *International Journal of Low Radiation*, 11(3/4), 186–206.
27. Kino K. (2024) Calculations of the radiation dose for the maximum hormesis effect. *Radiation*, 4(1), 69–84.
28. Feinendegen L.E. (1999) The role of adaptive responses following exposure to ionizing radiation. *Human & Experimental Toxicology*, 18(7).
29. Feinendegen L.E. (2005) Low doses of ionizing radiation: relationship between biological benefit and damage induction: a synopsis. *World Journal of Nuclear Medicine*, 4(1), 21–34.
30. Feinendegen L.E., Neumann R.D. (2005) Physics must join with biology in better assessing risk from low-dose irradiation. *Radiation Protection Dosimetry*, 117(4).
31. Feinendegen L.E. (2016) Quantification of adaptive protection following low-dose irradiation. *Health Physics*, 110(3), 276–280.
32. Feinendegen L.E., Pollycove M., Neumann R.D. (2007) New concepts in mammalian radiobiology. *Experimental Hematology*, 35, 37–46.
33. Fornalski K.W. (2016) Radiation and evolution: from Lotka-Volterra equation to balance equation. *International Journal of Low Radiation*, 10(3), 222–233.
34. Fornalski K.W. (2023) Application of Lotka-Volterra equations for homeostatic response to an ionizing radiation stressor. *Applied Sciences*, 13(11077).
35. Fornalski K.W. (2014) Mechanistic model of the cells irradiation using the stochastic biophysical input. *International Journal of Low Radiation*, 9(5/6), 370–395.
36. Fornalski K.W. (2022) Radioadaptation and radioresistance during deep space travels. *Journal of Space Safety Engineering*, (9)3, 385–389.
37. Fornalski K.W., Adamowski Ł., Dobrzyński L., Jarmakiewicz R., Powojska A., Reszczyńska J. (2022) The radiation adaptive response and priming dose influence: the quantification of the Raper-Yonezawa

effect and its three-parameter model for postradiation DNA lesions and mutations. *Radiation and Environmental Biophysics*, 61(7), 221–239.

38. Fornalski K.W., Adamowski Ł., Bugała E., Jarmakiewicz R., Krasowska J., Piotrowski Ł. (2024) Radiation adaptive response: the biophysical phenomenon and its theoretical description. Radiation Protection Dosimetry (accepted for publication). *NARE 2023 Conference Proceedings*, Special Issue.

Chapter 6

Low Background Radiations in Deep-Underground Environments

Jifeng Liu and Yuhao Zou
Deep Underground Space Medical Center and Department of Otolaryngology Head and Neck Surgery, West China Hospital, Sichuan University, China
liujifeng777@chscu.cn

Lives evolution has been influenced by natural background radiation on the Earth for about 4 billion years [1, 2]. Natural background radiation includes γ radiation, neutrons, muons, radon gas, and their daughter products in the rocks and atmosphere. The radiation level on our planet varies from 20 nGy/hr in underground spaces to 30 μGy/hr in the Ramsar region of Iran [3]. Hence, to what extent does natural radiation still confuse us. The linear no-threshold (LNT) is an assumption model, which assumes that the biological risk increases linearly under all radiation exposure without a threshold

Radioactivity in Life Sciences
Edited by Maria Letizia Terranova

ISBN 978-981-5129-67-0 (Hardcover), 978-1-003-63654-0 (eBook)
www.jennystanford.com

[4, 5]. However, an increasing number of researches conducted in deep-underground labs, which could dramatically shade cosmic radiation, have challenged this model [6]. Even, these studies showed that natural radiation was helpful for cells or organisms' homeostatic maintenance.

Deep-underground laboratories (DULs), divided into tunnel and underground types, were originally created to conduct nuclear physics experiments requiring an environment with reduced levels of cosmic ray particles by rock [7]. In 1964, Eugster's experiment observed cultures' behavior in DULs and began the biological experiment in DULs [8]. Since Prof. Sata transferred his interest from physics to biology of low background radiation (LBR) in the 1990s, a rising number of DULs worldwide provided more and more data on the biological response of cultures under the LBR in DULs [9]. The above knowledge is helpful for us to recognize the role of natural background radiation for life from a new perspective.

6.1 The Brief History of Biological Research in Deep-Underground Laboratories

The Simplon Pass with 2000 m rocky cover in the Swiss Alps was the first location, where the pioneering work investigating the biological effects of deep underground was conducted by Eugster in 1964 [8]. After about two decades, Planel et al. performed classical experiments at 200 m underground in Centre National de la Recherche Scientifique (CNRS) in Moulis of French Pyrenees [10]. Italy Gran Sasso National Laboratory (LNGS) with 1400 m rocky cover has conducted serial research on biological effects under LBR since 1995, when Satta et al. began their first study [9]. In 2011, Smith et al. conducted the first experiment in the Waste Isolation Pilot Plant (WIPP) in New Mexico, America, and explored the effects of LBR in the deep underground on living organisms [11]. In 2016, Lampe et al. published their LBR biological research conducted under a rocky cover of 1700 m in the Laboratory Souterrainde Modan (LSM) of the French Alps Fréjusroad Tunnel [12]. In 2017, Thome et al. published their LBR biological research program, which would be conducted at the Sudbury Neutrino Observatory (SNOLAB) with a depth of 2070 m in a nickel mine in Ontario, Canada [13]. In the same year, Prof. Xie et al. established a deep-underground laboratory in the Erdaogou Mine Jiapigou of Minerals Limited Corporation of China National Gold Group Corporation (CJEM), which focused on the biological effect in deep-underground with a depth of 1450 m [5]. In 2020, Pirkkanen and Wadsworth et al. published their research, respectively, conducted under LBR in Sudbury Neutrino Observatory Laboratory (SNOLAB) of Canada and Boulby Lab in England [14]. In 2021, Zarubi et al. first reported their research conducted DULB-4900 in the Baksan Neutrino Observatory with a rocky covey of 1800 m in Russia [15]. In 2022, China Jinping Deep Underground Lab (CJPL) with the lowest background radiation launched their biological project [16]. As of now, 13 DULs worldwide have or are engaged in biological research to elucidate the LBR influence on living systems in the deep-underground labs.

Besides, the Deep Underground Science and Engineering Laboratory (DUSEL) in Henderson Mine underground 2250 m near Empire, Colorado, had proposed a research project that aimed to investigate the biological effects of LBR in the deep-underground environment in 2011 [17]. In 2015, the ANDES underground laboratory with a rocky cover of 1800 m in the road tunnels of the Andes mountains in Argentina, the only underground laboratory in the Southern Hemisphere, announced the biological project focusing on the LBR underground [18]. The worldwide locations of DULs focusing on biological research of LBR are summarized in Fig. 6.1 and shown in Table 6.1.

[SIMP, Simplon Pass; WIPP, Waste Isolation Pilot Plant; CJEML, Laboratory of Jiapigou Minerals Limited Corporation of China National Gold Group Corporation; CJPL, Chinese Jinping Deep Underground Laboratory; DUSEL, Dusseldorf Underground Laboratory, USA; LNGS, Gran Sasso National Laboratory; DULB-4900, Baksan Neutrino Observatory; CNRS, Centre National de la Recherche Scientifique; ANDES, Argentina Agua Negra Extremely Deep Underground Laboratory; SNOLAB, Sudbury Neutrino Observatory Laboratory.]

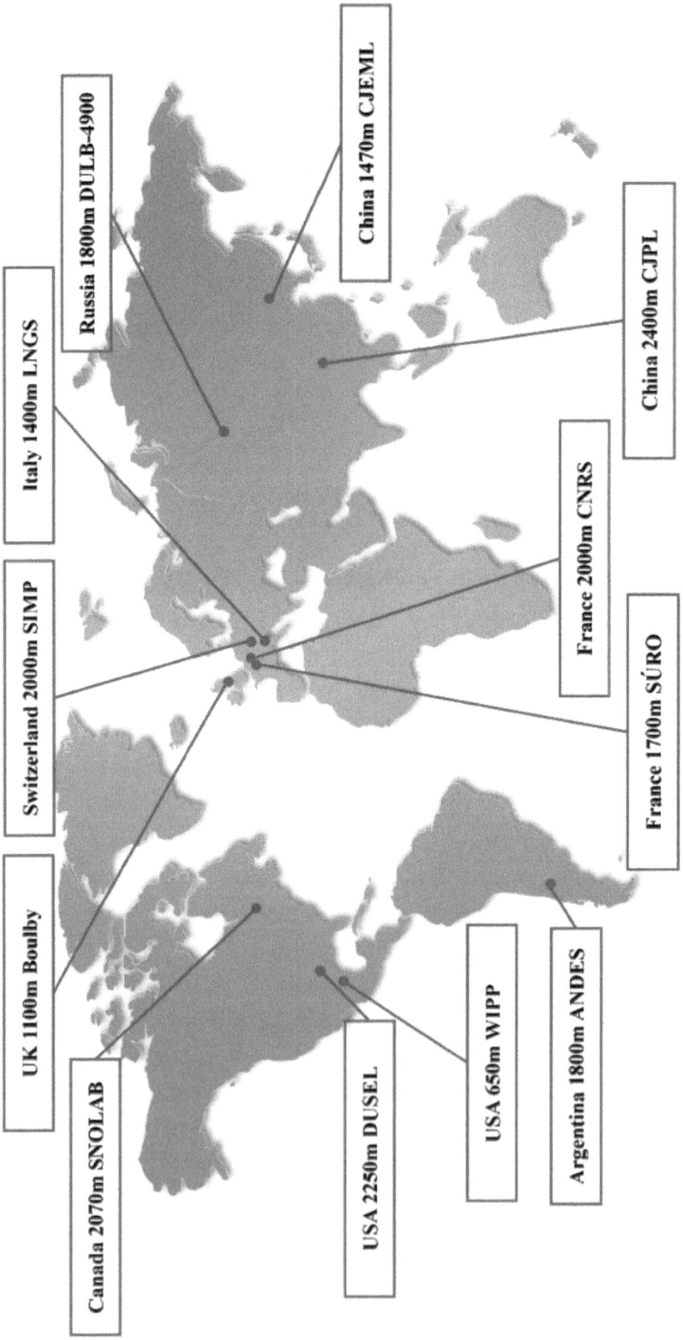

Figure 6.1 The location of DUGLs conducting biological research.

Table 6.1 The different biological effects of low background radiation on different organisms

Ref.	Laboratory	Depth (m)	Time	Value of radiation dose (LBR vs. CBR) (nGy/h)	Culture	Impact
[8]	SIMP	2000	A few weeks	Not stated	*Mastigogladus* I.	Died
[10]	CNRS	200 + 5 cm lead	10 days	11.4 vs 188.4	*Paramecium tetraurelia*	Growth↓
[11]	WIPP	650	75 h	2 vs 31	*Deinococcus radiodurans*	Growth↓, HSP70↑
[19]	WIPP	650	72 h	2 vs 31	*Shewanella oneidensis* *Deinococcus radiodurans*	Growth↓, KatB↑, SOA0154 ↑, RecA↑, Dps ↓, GAPDH↓, DnaK↑
[20]	WIPP	650	77 h	2 vs 31	*Deinococcus radiodurans*	Growth↓, DnaK↑
[21]	WIPP	605	34 h	0.91 vs 72.1	*Deinococcus radiodurans*	Growth↓, protein synthesis↓

(*Continued*)

Table 6.1 (*Continued*)

Ref.	Laboratory	Depth (m)	Time	Value of radiation dose (LBR vs. CBR) (nGy/h)	Culture	Impact
[22]	Boulby	1100	7 days	0.5 vs 112.5	*Bacillus subtilis, Escherichia coli*	Growth (-)
[23]	CJEM	1470	7 days	40 vs 150	V79	Growth↓, mitochondrial volume↑, hypertrophic ER, ribosomal and spliceosomal protein pathway enrichment, oxidoreductase↓, UQCRH↑, ATP6V1G1↑, DNA metabolic changes
[24]	CJEM	1470	4 days	40 vs 150	FD-LSC-1	Growth↓, ribosomal and spliceosomal protein pathway enrichment, mitochondrial volume↑, hypertrophic ER, UQCRH↑, ATP6V1G1↑, DNA metabolic changes
[25]	LNGS	1400	9 months	22 vs 122	V79	Growth (-), GST (-), SOD↓, HPRT mutation↑

Ref.	Laboratory	Depth (m)	Time	Value of radiation dose (LBR vs. CBR) (nGy/h)	Culture	Impact
[26]	WIPP	650	23 days	0.91 (LB) vs 35 (CB) vs 72 (UB)	V79	Viability↓, transcription-related genes↓
[27]	LNGS	1400	6 months	3.8 vs 331.7	TK6	Growth (-), SOD↓, GSH-PX↓, CAT↓,
[28]	WIPP	640	4 days	0.16 vs 71	*Shewanella oneidensis*	Growth (-), protein synthesis↓
[29]	LNGS	1400	9 months	22 vs 122	*Drosophila melanogaster*	Lifespan↑; fertility↓
[30]	WIPP	650	8 months	15.6 vs 67.4	*Caenorhabditis elegans* Nematode	Growth↑, egg-laying↑
[14]	SNOLAB	2000	4 months	11.55 vs 68.04	Lake Whitefish	Growth↑
[31]	CJEM	1470	2 days	40 vs 150	V79	Growth↓, RNA metabolic changes
[32]	LNGS	1400	5 generations	22 vs 122	*Drosophila melanogaster*	Chromosome breaks↑

(*Continued*)

Table 6.1 (*Continued*)

Ref.	Laboratory	Depth (m)	Time	Value of radiation dose (LBR vs. CBR) (nGy/h)	Culture	Impact
[33]	LNGS	1400	8months	22 vs 122	V79	SOD, CAT, GSH-PX, GSSG-RX, GST change
[34]	LNGS	1400	10 months	22.8 vs 94.7	V79	GSH-Px↓, HPRT mutation↑
[35]	LNGS	1400	1 month	22 vs 122	pKZ1 A11 mouse hybridoma cells	Growth (-), SOD↓, GSH-PX↓, CAT↓, Autophagy↑

SIMP, Simplon pass; CNRS, Centre National de la Recherche Scientifique; LNGS, the Gran Sasso National Laboratory; WIPP, Waste Isolation Pilot Plant; SNOLAB, Sudbury Neutrino Observatory Laboratory; CJEML, Laboratory of Jiapigou Minerals Limited Corporation of China National Gold Group Corporation; LBR, low background radiation; CBR, control background radiation; UB, underground background contains K-40; ER, endoplasmic reticulum; UQCRH, ubiquinol cytochrome c reductase hinge; ATP6V1G1, ATPase H+ Transporting V1 Subunit G1; SOD, superoxide dismutase; CAT, catalase; GST, glutathione transferase; GSSG-PX, glutathione peroxidase; GSSG-RX, glutathione reductase; HPRT, hypoxanthine guanine phosphoribosyl transfers.

6.2 The Environmental Characteristics of Deep-Underground Labs

Natural background radiation is composed of γ radiation, muons, neutrons, and radon gas. The γ radiation of DULs mainly originates from the rocks and atmosphere's 222Rn, 220Rn, and their daughter products [36]. The total background radiation level in DULs is only 1/5–1/10 of the control laboratories above ground (Table 6.1). Neutron flux comes from the decay of uranium and thorium in rocks and/or building materials and is very low in DULs [37]. Muons produced by the interaction of cosmic radiation with the Earth's atmosphere are effectively shielded by the rock of the DULs. The alpha particles come from the decay of radon gas released into the air [38].

In addition to LBR, the other environmental parameters should not be neglected, such as temperature, humidity, and air pressure. These factors are different from the above-ground environment. Watson et al. showed that the temperature in deep-underground mines increased by 3–5 °C per 100 m with increasing depth [39]. Relative humidity and air pressure also rise with increasing depth [40]. Liu et al. found that the humidity exceeds 90% at a depth of 600 m in the Erdaogou mine of Jiapigou Minerals Limited Corporation of China National Gold Group Corporation (CJEM) and the China Pingmei Shenma Group (CPSG) mine, which exceeds the acceptable maximum relative humidity for humans (70%) [41, 42]. Carbon dioxide and oxygen concentrations in the CJEM and CPSG are similar to above ground, due to appropriate ventilation [41, 42].

6.3 Biological Research under LBR in Deep-Underground Environment

The rocky cover of DULs can drastically shield cosmical rays and neutrons, so the DULs could provide a unique environment for investigating the biological effects of LBR. Hence, the research conducted in DULs mainly focuses on the biological effect of LBR. The increasing number of studies showed that the LBR has an obvious impact on organisms.

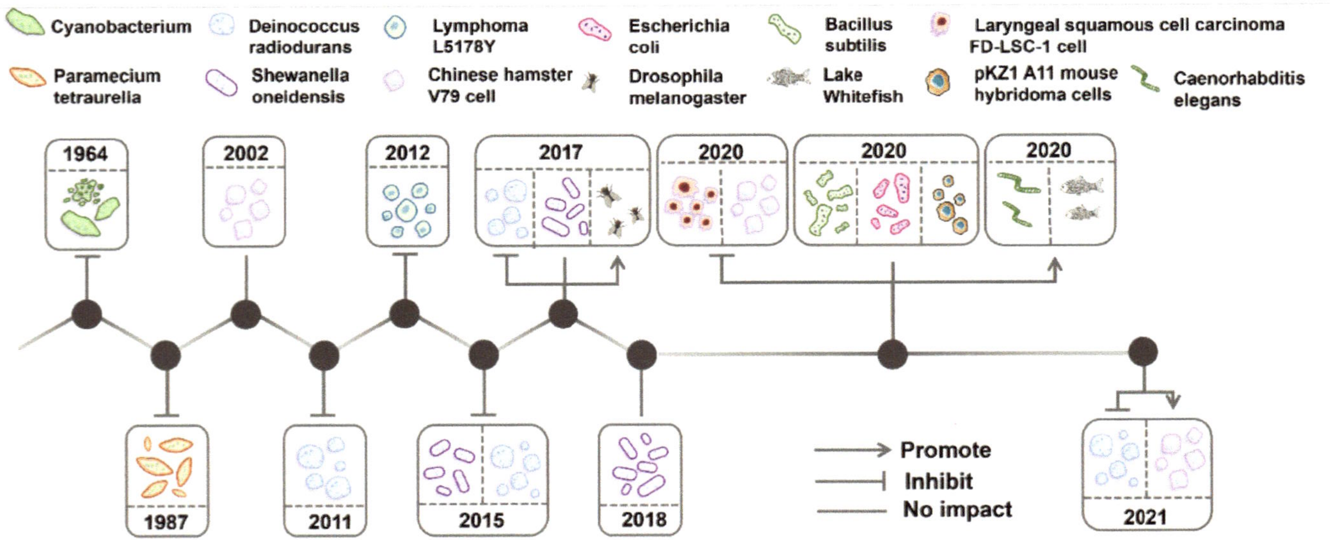

Figure 6.2 Low background radiation in deep-underground laboratories affects the growth of living organisms. The impacts of LBR in the DUGE on the growth patterns of single-celled and multicellular organisms.

6.3.1 The Growth of Organisms under LBR Environment

In 1964, the pioneer biological work in DULs conducted by Eugster showed that the cyanobacterium *Mastigocladus laminosus* cultured in the Simplon Tunnel (2000 m of rock cover) died after a few weeks [8] (Fig. 6.2). However, this study did not describe the background radiation value in Simplon Tunnel. In 1987, Planel et al. published their classical research on the LBR biological effect, which showed that the *Paramecium tetraurelia* cultures grown in the underground laboratory at the CNRS had reduced cell number and increased generation time [10]. The enhanced inhibitory effect was observed when the cultures were further shielded from exposure to underground radiation by 5 cm of old lead. In contrast, the *Paramecium tetraurelia* proliferation increased when they were cultured under high background radiation in highlands and space stations [10]. In 2011, Smith et al. presented compelling evidence for reduced growth rates in *Deinococcus radiodurans* cultures grown 650 m below ground in a pre-World War II steel chamber at the WIPP compared to parallel populations cultured above ground [11]. Further support for this phenomenon was provided by Castillo et al., who showed growth rates of both *Shewanella oneidensis* and *D. radiodurans* cultures were reduced within 24 h culture in WIPP compared to parallel populations grown in the same laboratory with a simulated standard background environment [19, 20]. A similar occurrence was also confirmed by Kawanishi et al., who incubated mouse lymphoma L5178Y cells in a shielded chamber surrounded by a 15 cm thick iron wall and a 10 cm thick paraffin wall that could reduce the γ-ray and neutron levels in the chamber to 2% and 25% of the background levels, respectively [43].

However, human lymphoblastoid TK6, Chinese hamster V79, and pKZ1 A11 mouse hybridoma cells did not present a clear difference in growth rates between cells, respectively, cultured in the control environment above ground and in the LBR environment of LNGS for several weeks to months [25, 27, 35]. Similarly, Castillo et al. did not show that growth rates were affected when *Shewanella oneidensis* was cultured in the WIPP [28, 44]. Satta et al. found that V79 cells cultured in LNGS for 9 months grew normally, and Wadsworth et al. showed that growth rates of *Bacillus subtilis* and *Escherichia coli* had no obvious change after 7 days of incubation in Boulby Lab [22, 25]. Even, Castillo et al. discovered that V79 cells cultured for 23 days under the LBR in the WIPP had a higher and more variable number of cells and more heterogeneous cell populations compared to those grown above ground [26]. Hence, the growth rate of cells under the LBR environment is still controversial. To confirm whether LBR could inhibit cell growth, Liu et al. conducted serial studies in CJEM and China Jinping Underground Laboratory (CJPL) at different times and confirmed this inhibition phenomenon by studying the mammalian cell growth rates [23, 24]. Fortunately, the inhibition growth rates of the single-celled organisms cultured in the LBR of DULs could be rescued by the introduction of an exogenous simulated radiation source [11, 43].

In recent years, research about LBR biological effects conducted in DULs has extended to multicellular organisms. Morciano et al. first cultured *Drosophila melanogaster* in LNGS and found an increased lifespan but decreased fertility of adult males and females [29]. *D. melanogaster* cultured for five generations in LBR of LNGS showed a stress response and chromosomal damage with a cross-generational effect [32]. Van Voorhies et al. found that *Caenorhabditis elegans*' egg-laying rates and larval growth were increased when exposed to LBR in WIPP compared to normal background radiation levels [30]. Pirkkanen et al. cultured Lake Whitefish under LBR in SNOLAB and showed no significant differences in hatching time or survival rates between the experiment and control group [14]. However, embryos raised underground were larger than the above-ground control group. The authors speculated that higher radon levels underground (100–150 Bq/m^3) stimulated embryos reared in the SNOLAB with significantly larger body sizes [13].

Although the different organisms maintained in the LBR of DULs exhibit different changes in growth, the single-celled organisms presented with growth inhibition in a short time can be confirmed. Whereas a few research about multicellular cultures and long-time observation for single-celled organisms under the LBR environment limited us to getting a solid conclusion, this suggested that more types and longer-term investigations about cultures' response under the LBR still need to be conducted in the future [45].

6.3.2 The Change of Organelles of Organisms under the LBR Environment

With a double-membrane system, mitochondria are an energy-providing organelle for the activities of eukaryotic cells [46]. Mitochondria play an important role in stress response. Mitochondrial reactive oxygen species (ROS) produced in physiological and pathological conditions can induce damage to cells [47, 48]. Liu et al. found that mitochondrial volume increased and mitochondria cristae decreased in V79 cells and FD-LSC-1 cells cultured in CJEM compared to the cells cultured above ground [23, 24]. These findings were further confirmed in thyroid epithelial cells, which were very sensitive to radiation. Besides, our recent work conducted in CJPL also observed the morphological change of cells cultured in the LBR.

The endoplasmic reticulum (ER), a direct intracellular target of radiation, is highly sensitive to changes in the external environment [49]. Mild ER stress initiates autophagy to maintain ER homeostasis and protect cells from damage [50]. Liu et al. showed that V79 and FD-LSC-1 cells cultured under the LBR in CEJM presented hypertrophic ER, obvious Golgi bodies, and downregulation of major ER stress proteins (WFS1, STT3B, CANX, ERP29, and HSPA5) compared to cells cultured above ground [23, 24]. Transcriptomics demonstrated that differently expressed (DE) circRNAs between V79 cells cultured in the DULs and above-ground labs were predominantly enriched in protein processing in the ER [31].

Ribosomes play an important role in protein translation and cell proliferation [51]. Castillo et al. found that the ribosomal proteins and tRNA genes in *S. oneidensis* deprived of background radiation were down-regulated, which indicated an obvious decrease in protein translation [28]. A similar phenomenon was verified by Liu et al., who showed changes in protein expression associated with the ribosome pathway in V79 and FD-LSC-1 cells cultured in the LBR of CJEM compared to the control group above ground. KEGG enrichment analysis of DE proteins also showed that ribosome biogenesis and ribosomal proteins (such as RPS6, RPS14, RPS16, RPL8, RPL23, RPL3, and RPS18) played a key role in the regulation of cell growth for cells under the LBR in DUL [23, 24].

Spliceosomes, regulating gene expression and protein synthesis, are essential organelles for cell growth and division [52]. Liu et al. found DE proteins of V79 and FD-LSC-1 cells between cultures in CJEM and above ground. Besides, DE LncRNAs of V79 cells were significantly enriched in the spliceosome pathway [23, 24, 31].

Briefly, although the research conducted on the LBR in DULs is still limited, these data imply that mitochondria, ER, ribosomes, and the spliceosome are involved in the stress and adaptive responses of cells exposed to LBR in the deep-underground environment. However, the potential mechanism underlying the role of these organelles for cells' response to LBR in a deep-underground environment requires further research.

6.3.3 LBR Induces Organisms Stress Response in Molecular Level

6.3.3.1 Oxidative stress

Oxidative stress is an important progress in stress response, especially for radiation exposure. Therefore, the initial series of biological research on LBR conducted in LNGS focused on oxidative stress. Antonelli et al. found the activity changes of antioxidant enzymes (superoxide dismutase [SOD], catalase [CAT], glutathione peroxidase, reductase, and transferase [GSH-PX, GSSG-RX, GST]) of V79 cells grown in the LNGS [33]. Satta et al. further showed that the SOD activity of V79 cells cultured in LBR was lower than those in the standard environment for 9 months, while the GST activity was at the same level between the two groups [25]. Carbone et al. also found that SOD, GSH-PX, CATase, CAT/SOD activity, and SE-GSH-PX/SOD ratios decreased in human lymphoblastoid TK6 cells cultured in LNGS compared to these in the reference environmental radiation conditions [27]. Meanwhile, Fratini et al. found GSH-Px activity in V79 cells also decreased, when they were cultured for 10 months in LNGS [34]. This change did not revert to a normal state when the cells were brought back to the reference-radiation environment even after 6 months.

In WIPP, a similar phenomenon was observed. Castillo et al. demonstrated that the oxidative stress-related genes katB and SOA0154 and the DNA damage-related gene recA were upregulated in *S. oneidensis*, while dps (DNA protection against ROS) and gapd H (ATP synthesis) genes were downregulated in *Deinococcus radiodurans* incubated in LBR of WIPP for 76 h compared to background radiation control group [19]. Furthermore, Smith et al. also observed the upregulation of heat shock protein 70 (HSP70) in primary human lung fibroblasts and bronchial epithelial cells cultured in reduced radiation levels in WIPP compared to the control background [11].

Omic analyses are helpful in understanding the molecular change of organisms from the whole perspective. Liu et al. performed the whole proteomic and transcriptomic analyses to reveal the molecular response of V79 and FD-LSC-1 cells under the LBR in CJEM [23, 24]. The two cell lines cultured under the LBR in CJEM showed that many down-regulated proteins enriched in oxidoreductase activity and the redox process, while ubiquinol cytochrome c reductase hinge (UQCRH) and ATPase H+ Transporting V1 Subunit G1 (ATP6V1G1) of cells in the LBR group upregulated [23, 24]. As to transcriptomic level, the DE mRNAs between V79 cells cultured in the DUL and above-ground control lab were mainly enriched in redox activity and redox processes, and the DE mRNAs of FD-LSC-1 cells were also enriched in SOD-related entities [31].

Taken together, these data from different labs implied that LBR in the deep-underground environment could induce cells' change of oxidative stress. However, the core mechanism and target factors remain to be elucidated in the future.

6.3.3.2 The defense response against external factors

Satta et al. found *S cerevisiae* D7 exposed to recombinogenic doses of methyl methane sulfonate grown in the LBR compared to a standard environment presented a higher frequency of radiomimetic-induced recombination [9]. A subsequent study showed that V79 cells grown in reduced environmental radiation conditions for 9 months were more susceptible to cycloheximide-induced apoptosis and had an increased frequency of mutations of the hypoxanthine-guanine phosphoribosyl transferase (HPRT) gene induced by γ-ray exposure compared to cells grown in a standard background environment [25]. Similarly, Fratini et al. and Antonelli et al. observed an increased rate of spontaneous HPRT mutations in V79 cells cultured in the LBR [33, 34]. Carbone et al. [27, 53] demonstrated that the level of DNA damage and repair and management of ROS balance was different in TK6 cells exposed to 2Gy X-ray irradiation in a DUL compared to a standard environment for 6 months. Castillo et al. [19, 20] showed upregulation of dnaK in *D. radiodurans* cultured in the LBR compared to normal background radiation. This change was also confirmed in the multicellular organism *Drosophila Oregon R (OR-R)* line. Porrazzo et al. showed that the reduced radiation background in the LNGS underground laboratory rendered *Drosophila* neuroblasts more sensitive to ionizing radiation-induced DNA breaks compared to fruit flies cultured at the external reference laboratory [32]. This damage could be rescued by increasing the underground gamma dose rate to levels comparable to the reference radiation level.

All in all, these previous researches implied that deprivation of natural levels of environmental radiation might increase the frequency of gene recombination and susceptibility of cells to damaging factors. In other words, the background radiation might be beneficial for the steady-state maintenance of organisms.

6.3.3.3 Metabolic responses

Organisms' metabolic processes exposed to LBR have been affected, which covers DNA, RNA, and proteins. Castillo et al. found that the protein synthesis of *D. radiodurans* exposed to LBR was inhibited, which presented with a decreased number of ribosomes, downregulation of tRNA, and transcription of HSP genes [21, 28]. In their following study, Castillo et al. also showed that V79 cells' transcription-related mRNAs were downregulated when they were cultured in LBR of WIPP [26]. Liu and his team's series of works conducted in CJEM had the same result. Their research revealed that the RNA profile altered compared to the control when V79 and FD-LSC-1 cells were cultured in the LBR in CJEM, which had negative impacts on metabolic processes [31, 54]. Also, the changes involved in modifications of DNA replication, transcription, translation, and protein modification. Liu et al. also revealed that the DE RNAs of FD-LSC-1 cells were cultured in LBR in CJEM enriched in TGF-β and Hippo signaling pathway, the late pathway is a pathway related to proliferation inhibition induced by environmental stimulation [23, 24]. Besides, the expression of proliferation genes SMAD, SMAD7, CDH1, EGR1, and BMP2 of FD-LSC-1 changed significantly, which showed that these genes played key roles in the transcriptional regulation of FD-LSC-1 cells under LBR environmental stress [55].

Autophagy is an important biological progress involved in many physiological and pathological mechanisms. Fischietti et al. found that pKZ1 A11 mouse hybridoma cells in the LBR condition responded to growth stress by switching toward autophagy, this was different from cells triggering apoptosis under the same stress in normal background radiation conditions [35]. Also, this research showed that this response was not caused by the γ component.

Together, these data imply that cells can perceive LBR in the deep-underground environment and generate stress responses, resulting in changes in metabolic processes at different molecular levels.

6.4 The Effect of Deep-Underground Environment on Human

As resources and space in shallow earth have become exhausted, many countries have aimed to explore and exploit the deep underground. Therefore, an increasing number of people will live and work in the deep-underground space in the future, and it is necessary to reveal the effect of the deep-underground environment on human pathology, psychology, and physiology. Even, Prof. Xie advocated the need for a new multidisciplinary, deep-underground medicine (DUGM) approach to cope with this situation.

Some researchers have focused on the deep-underground environmental effect on humans. Strzemecka et al. [40] surveyed 700 miners working underground in the Bogdanka Coal Mine at a depth of 1100 m and revealed that 50% of them perceived the microclimate in the mine, such as high humidity and temperatures, threatening their health (Fig. 6.3). Meshi et al. reported that 78.4% of miners of the Mara Gold Mine in Tanzania suffered from moderate heat-related illness, such as high body temperature, hot and dry skin. The mine, located at a depth of 500 m in the tropics, has an ambient temperature of 28.4 °C and relative humidity of over 58.2% [56]. Liu et al. surveyed the subjective perceptions and mental state of employees of CJEM (1470 m) and CPSG (1500 m), respectively, and

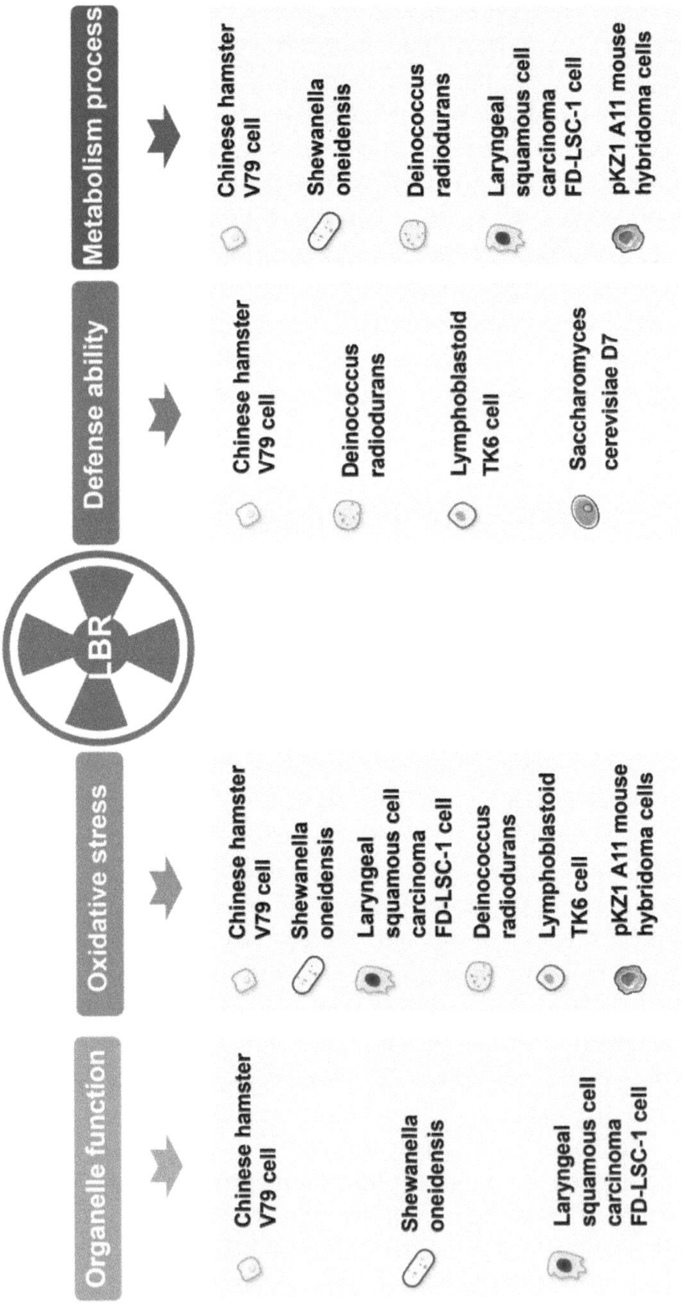

Figure 6.3 Cellular responses to low background radiation in deep-underground laboratories.

showed that moisture and heat were the most commonly perceived adverse factors in the deep-underground spaces [41, 42]. Also, Liu et al. investigated the mental state of 496 miners who worked at a depth below 600 m in the CJEM and CPSG [57–59]. These miners at both mines complained of being easily fatigued, having trouble sleeping, and waking up early in the morning. Meanwhile, Wen et al. performed urine metabolomics analysis of miners and indicated that the deep-underground environment induces specific changes in the metabolism of amino acids (L-phenylalanine, L-tyrosine, and L-glutamine) in humans, and these changes were helpful in explaining the sleep disorders of miners in the deep earth [16].

Although the LBR is a unique environmental character in the deep underground and can be perceived by cells, it is not easy to bring about obvious effects in humans. Notley, this does not mean that LBR has no effect on humans. In other words, this might be covered by other environmental factors, such as high temperature and humanity. Therefore, it is necessary to detect LBR's short and long-term effects on humans under control conditions.

The low background radiation can induce a stress response and affect the organelles' function, defense capacity, oxidative stress, and metabolism of cells.

6.5 Conclusions

The utilization and exploitation of deep-underground resources and space have become a national strategy for many developed countries. However, previous research suggested that the unique LBR factor in the deep-underground environment could induce a stress response in living organisms. Mitochondria, ER, ribosomes, spliceosomes, etc. might be the responsible organelles for the stress response of cells cultured in an LBR environment. Meanwhile, the unique environmental factor might have a potential effect on humans, especially for amino acid metabolism. However, the interconnections and feedback regulation of organisms between organelles and underlying molecular mechanisms remain unclear. Meanwhile, it does not mean all these responses have harmful effects on organisms. For example, our previous research showed that LBR in the deep-underground environment had an inhibitory effect on the proliferation of cancer cells, especially for radiation-sensitive cancer cells, which might provide a potentially new perspective for cancer control. Currently, knowledge about LBR in deep-underground environments is still limited, which will limit the step to deep earth. In the future, it is necessary to explore the biological effects of LBR in the deep-underground environment on living systems.

DULs own a unique clear radiation background and could provide a platform for detecting the biological effects of various components of radiation (radon gas, γ, etc.) and their dose responses. Previous studies have shown that the deep-underground environment affected human pathology, psychology, and physiology. However, except for LBR, the environmental factors in the deep-underground environment involve many components, such as rock components, humidity, temperature, illumination, and other unknown factors. Therefore, it is necessary to qualitatively and quantitatively characterize the environmental factors in the deep-underground environment and illustrate their potential beneficial and adverse effects on humans. So that we could inform strategies that facilitate human adaptation and habituation to the deep-underground environment. Notably, the long-term consequences of exposure to factors in the deep-underground environment in humans must be monitored, and cross-disciplinary research between deep-underground medicine and various clinical disciplines is required to support sustained development and utilization of the deep-underground space.

References

1. UNSCEAR, 2000 Report to the General Assembly with Scientific Annexes. *Sources*, 2001.
2. Belli, M. and L. Indovina, The response of living organisms to low radiation environment and its implications in radiation protection. *Front Public Health*, 2020. **8**: p. 601711.
3. Welsh, J.S., J.J. Bevelacqua, and S.M.J. Mortazavi, Ramsar, Iran, as a natural radiobiological surrogate for mars. *Health Phys*, 2022. **122**(4): p. 508–512.
4. UNSCEAR, *Biological Mechanisms of Radiation Actions at Low Doses.* New York, NY: United Nations, 2012.

5. Liu, J., et al., History, advancements, and perspective of biological research in deep-underground laboratories: a brief review. *Environ Int*, 2018. **120**: p. 207–214.
6. Adelstein, S.J., Biologic responses to low doses of ionizing radiation: adaptive response versus bystander effect. *J Nucl Med*, 2003. **44**(1): p. 125; author reply 125–126.
7. Laubenstein, M. and I. Lawson, Low background radiation detection techniques and mitigation of radioactive backgrounds. *Frontiers in Physics*, 2020. **8**.
8. Eugster, J.G., Subradiation experiments concerning the concept of the natural radiation environment. *Aerosp Med*, 1964. **35**: p. 524–526.
9. Satta, L., et al., Low environmental radiation background impairs biological defence of the yeast Saccharomyces cerevisiae to chemical radiomimetic agents. *Mutat Res*, 1995. **347**(3–4): p. 129–133.
10. Planel, H., et al., Influence on cell proliferation of background radiation or exposure to very low, chronic gamma radiation. *Health Physics*, 1987. **52**(5): p. 571–578.
11. Smith, G.B., et al., Exploring biological effects of low level radiation from the other side of background. *Health Phys*, 2011. **100**(3): p. 263–265.
12. Lampe, N., et al., Simulating the impact of the natural radiation background on bacterial systems: implications for very low radiation biological experiments. *PLoS One*, 2016. **11**(11): p. e0166364.
13. Thome, C., et al., Initial characterization of the growth stimulation and heat-shock-induced adaptive response in developing lake whitefish embryos after ionizing radiation exposure. *Radiat Res*, 2017. **188**(4.2): p. 475–485.
14. Pirkkanen, J., et al., A Research environment 2 km deep-underground impacts embryonic development in Lake Whitefish (Coregonus clupeaformis). *Frontiers in Earth Science*, 2020. **8**.
15. Zarubin, M., et al., First transcriptome profiling of D. melanogaster after development in a deep underground low radiation background laboratory. *PLoS One*, 2021. **16**(8): p. e0255066.
16. Wen, Q., et al., Urine metabolomics analysis of sleep quality in deep-underground miners: a pilot study. *Frontiers in Public Health*, 2022. **10**.
17. Jung, C.K., Henderson deep underground science and engineering lab: unearthing the secrets of the universe, underground. *Nuclear Physics B - Proceedings Supplements*, 2011. **221**: p. 125–129.

18. Civitarese, O., The ANDES underground laboratory project. *Nuclear and Particle Physics Proceedings*, 2015. **267–269**: p. 377–381.

19. Castillo, H., et al., Stress induction in the bacteria Shewanella oneidensis and Deinococcus radiodurans in response to below-background ionizing radiation. *Int J Radiat Biol*, 2015. **91**(9): p. 749–756.

20. Castillo, H. and G.B. Smith, Below-background ionizing radiation as an environmental cue for bacteria. *Frontiers in Microbiology*, 2017. **8**.

21. Castillo, H., X. Li, and G.B. Smith, Deinococcus radiodurans UWO298 dependence on background radiation for optimal growth. *Front Genet*, 2021. **12**: p. 644292.

22. Wadsworth, J., et al., There's plenty of room at the bottom: low radiation as a biological extreme. *Frontiers in Astronomy and Space Sciences*, 2020. **7**.

23. Liu, J., et al., Proteomics provides insights into the inhibition of Chinese hamster V79 cell proliferation in the deep underground environment. *Sci Rep*, 2020. **10**(1): p. 14921.

24. Liu, J., et al., Proteomic characterization of proliferation inhibition of well-differentiated laryngeal squamous cell carcinoma cells under below-background radiation in a deep underground environment. *Front Public Health*, 2020. **8**: p. 584964.

25. Satta, L., et al., Influence of a low background radiation environment on biochemical and biological responses in V79 cells. *Radiat Environ Biophys*, 2002. **41**(3): p. 217–224.

26. Castillo, H., J. Winder, and G. Smith, Chinese hamster V79 cells' dependence on background ionizing radiation for optimal growth. *Radiat Environ Biophys*, 2022. **61**(1): p. 49–57.

27. Carbone, M.C., et al., The cosmic silence experiment: on the putative adaptive role of environmental ionizing radiation. *Radiat Environ Biophys*, 2009. **48**(2): p. 189–196.

28. Castillo, H., et al., Transcriptome analysis reveals a stress response of Shewanella oneidensis deprived of background levels of ionizing radiation. *PLoS One*, 2018. **13**(5): p. e0196472.

29. Morciano, P., et al., Effects of reduced natural background radiation on Drosophila melanogaster growth and development as revealed by the FLYINGLOW program. *J Cell Physiol*, 2018. **233**(1): p. 23–29.

30. Van Voorhies, W.A., et al., The phenotypic and transcriptomic response of the Caenorhabditis elegans nematode to background and below-background radiation levels. *Front Public Health*, 2020. **8**: p. 581796.

31. Duan, L., et al., Whole transcriptome analysis revealed a stress response to deep underground environment conditions in Chinese Hamster V79 lung fibroblast cells. *Front Genet*, 2021. **12**: p. 698046.

32. Porrazzo, A., et al., Reduced environmental dose rates are responsible for the increased susceptibility to radiation-induced DNA damage in larval neuroblasts of drosophila grown inside the LNGS underground laboratory. *Int J Mol Sci*, 2022. **23**(10).

33. Antonelli, F., et al., Radiation biophysics at the Gran Sasso laboratory: influence of a low background radiation environment on the adaptive response of living cells. *Nuclear Physics B - Proceedings Supplements*, 2000. **87**(1–3): p. 508–509.

34. Fratini, E., et al., Low-radiation environment affects the development of protection mechanisms in V79 cells. *Radiat Environ Biophys*, 2015. **54**(2): p. 183–194.

35. Fischietti, M., et al., Low radiation environment switches the overgrowth-induced cell apoptosis toward autophagy. *Front Public Health*, 2020. **8**: p. 594789.

36. Morciano, P., et al., Fruit flies provide new insights in low-radiation background biology at the INFN Underground Gran Sasso National Laboratory (LNGS). *Radiat Res*, 2018. **190**(3): p. 217–225.

37. Zarubin, M.P., O.A. Kuldoshina, and E.V. Kravchenko, Biological effects of low background radiation: prospects for future research in the low-background laboratory DULB-4900 of Baksan Neutrino Observatory INR RAS. *Physics of Particles and Nuclei*, 2021. **52**(1): p. 19–30.

38. Bacioiu, I., Equivalent dose rate by muons to the human body. *Radiat Prot Dosimetry*, 2011. **147**(3): p. 380–385.

39. Watson, T.L., Underground temperatures. *Science*, 1911. **33**(856): p. 828–831.

40. Strzemecka, J., et al., Factors of work environment hazardous for health in opinions of employees working underground in the 'Bogdanka' coal mine. *Ann Agric Environ Med*, 2019. **26**(3): p. 409–414.

41. Liu, J., et al., Subjective perceptions and psychological distress associated with the deep underground: a cross-sectional study in a deep gold mine in China. *Medicine (Baltimore)*, 2019. **98**(22): p. e15571.

42. Xie, H., et al., Physical symptoms and mental health status in deep underground miners: a cross-sectional study. *Medicine (Baltimore)*, 2020. **99**(9): p. e19294.

43. Kawanishi, M., et al., Growth retardation of Paramecium and mouse cells by shielding them from background radiation. *J Radiat Res*, 2012. **53**(3): p. 404–410.

44. Hugo, C. and G.B. Smith, Below-Background Ionizing Radiation as an environmental cue for bacteria. *Frontiers in Microbiology*, 2017. **8**.

45. Daly, M.J., et al., Accumulation of Mn(II) in Deinococcus radiodurans facilitates gamma-radiation resistance. *Science*, 2004. **306**(5698): p. 1025–1028.

46. Lu, Z., et al., iTRAQ-based proteomic analysis on the mitochondrial responses in gill tissues of juvenile olive flounder Paralichthys olivaceus exposed to cadmium. *Environ Pollut*, 2020. **257**: p. 113591.

47. Napolitano, G., G. Fasciolo, and P. Venditti, Mitochondrial management of reactive oxygen species. *Antioxidants (Basel)*, 2021. **10**(11).

48. Wilson, D.F., Oxidative phosphorylation: regulation and role in cellular and tissue metabolism. *J Physiol*, 2017. **595**(23): p. 7023–7038.

49. Wang, J.S., H.J. Wang, and H.L. Qian, Biological effects of radiation on cancer cells. *Mil Med Res*, 2018. **5**(1): p. 20.

50. Scheper, W., D.A. Nijholt, and J.J. Hoozemans, The unfolded protein response and proteostasis in Alzheimer disease: preferential activation of autophagy by endoplasmic reticulum stress. *Autophagy*, 2011. **7**(8): p. 910–911.

51. Zhou, X., et al., Ribosomal proteins: functions beyond the ribosome. *J Mol Cell Biol*, 2015. **7**(2): p. 92–104.

52. Will, C.L. and R. Lührmann, Spliceosome structure and function. *Cold Spring Harb Perspect Biol*, 2011. **3**(7).

53. Carbone, M.C., et al., Effects of deprivation of background environmental radiation on cultured human cells. *Nuovo Cimento- Societa Italiana di Fisica Sezione B*, 2010. **125**(4): p. 469–477.

54. Liu, Y., et al., Transcriptome analysis of well-differentiated laryngeal squamous cell carcinoma cells in below-background environment. *Annals of Translational Medicine*, 2022. **10**(15): p. 824–824.

55. Liu, Y., et al., Transcriptome analysis of well-differentiated laryngeal squamous cell carcinoma cells in below-background environment. *Ann Transl Med*, 2022. **10**(15): p. 824.

56. Meshi, E.B., et al., Thermal exposure and heat illness symptoms among workers in Mara Gold Mine, Tanzania. *Ann Glob Health*, 2018. **84**(3): p. 360–368.

57. Liu, L., L. Wang, and J. Chen, Prevalence and associated factors of depressive symptoms among Chinese underground coal miners. *Biomed Res Int*, 2014. **2014**: p. 987305.

58. McLean, K.N., Mental health and well-being in resident mine workers: out of the fly-in fly-out box. *Aust J Rural Health*, 2012. **20**(3): p. 126–130.

59. Hristov, Z.I., Psychoemotional stress of employees and workers in the public and real sectors of national economy in Bulgaria. *Folia Med (Plovdiv)*, 2009. **51**(2): p. 58–67.

Chapter 7

Astronaut Health in Space: Bio-Defenses Against Radiation and Microgravity

Alireza Mortazavi,[a] SMJ Mortazavi,[b] Hassan Vafapour,[b] Razi Rashidfar,[b] Zeynab Seyeddi,[b] Najmeh Jooyan,[b] Fatemeh Bensaeid,[b] Lembit Sihver,[c,d] and James Welsh[e,f]

[a]*MVLS College, The University of Glasgow, Glasgow, Scotland, UK*

[b]*Ionizing and Non-ionizing Radiation Protection Research Center (INIRPRC), Shiraz University of Medical Sciences, Shiraz, Iran*

[c]*Department of Informatics & Engineering Systems, University of Texas Rio Grande Valley, TX, USA*

[d]*Department of Chemistry and Chemical Engineering, Royal Military College of Canada, Kingston, ON, Canada*

[e]*Department of Radiation Oncology, Edward Hines Jr VA Hospital, Hines, IL, USA*

[f]*Department of Radiation Oncology, Loyola University Stritch School of Medicine, Chicago, USA*

lembit.sihver@tuwien.ac.at, shermanwelsh@gmail.com

Astronauts venturing far beyond the Earth face a significant health hazard: radiation exposure. Current shielding provides some protection, but it is insufficient for the extended durations of deep

Radioactivity in Life Sciences
Edited by Maria Letizia Terranova

ISBN 978-981-5129-67-0 (Hardcover), 978-1-003-63654-0 (eBook)
www.jennystanford.com

space journeys. To enhance astronaut safety, scientists are actively developing new protective strategies. A promising approach involves pre-selecting astronauts based on their genetic predisposition for radiation tolerance. By assessing their radioadaptive response through in vitro cytogenetic tests before launch, we can identify individuals who are naturally more resistant to radiation. Additionally, the use of radioprotectors, which protect cells against space radiation, and radiomitigators, which reduce damage after exposure, could be essential. In specific scenarios, techniques such as induced hibernation or immune system enhancement might also be beneficial. Diet, too, plays a crucial role in safeguarding astronauts from radiation and the effects of microgravity. The potential role of physical and mental activities will also be explored in this chapter. In summary, extensive research is still required to refine these strategies and ensure their effectiveness for long-term space missions.

7.1 Introduction

Radiation exposure in space, particularly during long-duration missions beyond low Earth orbit (LEO), is a significant concern. The deep space environment exposes astronauts to galactic cosmic rays and solar radiation, which can have adverse effects on human health, including the risk of radiation sickness. Managing these health risks requires advanced medical capabilities and countermeasures. Incorporating expanded medical capabilities for treating radiation-induced illnesses would indeed require substantial research, time, and funding. The development of effective radiation protection strategies is essential to ensure the safety and health of astronauts during long-duration missions beyond LEO. The current methods of radiation protection for astronauts are mostly based on passive and active shielding. Passive shielding involves the use of physical materials to block or slow down energetic particles, while active shielding aims to mimic the Earth's magnetic field using superconducting magnets or localized electric or magnetic fields. However, biological protection methods, such as using natural radioprotectors are pharmacologic agents administered before radiation exposure to mitigate their effects, are of crucial importance.

Besides radioprotectors, mitigators can be administered after exposure to reduce the symptoms of radiation disease. Moreover, other methods including immune system modulators can be used to protect astronauts from the biological consequences of space radiation.

While current medical resources for spaceflight may address some aspects of radiation sickness, the unique conditions of space travel pose specific challenges that necessitate further research and development [1]. Some potential avenues for improvement include the development of advanced radiation shielding technologies, medical interventions to mitigate radiation effects, and improved diagnostic and treatment methods. Furthermore, the limitations of current spacecraft may pose challenges in implementing these enhanced medical capabilities. Spacecraft design constraints, mass limitations, and power considerations may limit the feasibility of carrying extensive medical equipment or establishing fully equipped medical facilities on exploration vehicles. Figure 7.1 shows some key biological strategies to support prolonged deep space explorations.

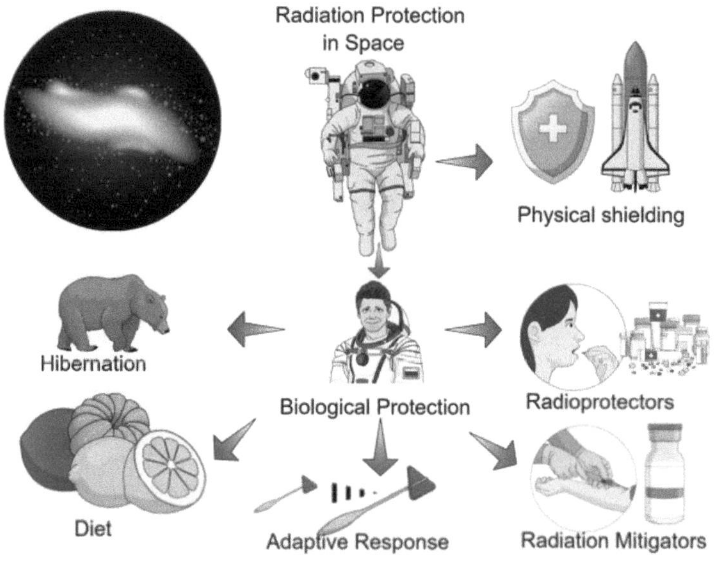

Figure 7.1 Some key biological strategies to support prolonged deep space explorations.

Therefore, ongoing research and development efforts are essential to advancing our understanding of the effects of space radiation and developing effective countermeasures to ensure the health and safety of astronauts during long-duration space missions. Addressing these challenges requires a multidisciplinary approach, involving collaboration between space agencies, medical researchers, engineers, and other relevant fields.

7.2 The Scope of the Problem

The current technology for radiation protection is not fully optimized, but it still provides significant protection for crews on Lunar or Mars design reference missions [2]. Passive and active shielding alone cannot sufficiently reduce the risks of radiation for long-term deep space missions [3]. It is crucial to develop alternative measures to mitigate the health risks associated with radiation. In addition to shielding, conducting pre-flight screening of candidates to assess their level of radio adaptation based on genetic differences could help reduce radiation-induced health risks [3]. Furthermore, advanced medical countermeasures such as radioprotectors and radiomitigators will likely be necessary in future deep space missions. Vitamin C has shown promise as a non-toxic, cost-effective, readily available radiation mitigator. Additionally, strategies like hibernation and boosting the immune system may be employed in specific circumstances. Diet also plays a critical role in protecting astronauts from radiation and microgravity. However, further research is necessary to develop and optimize radiation countermeasures for deep space missions. In the realm of space research and radiologic terrorism, a significant amount of attention has been directed toward the development of strategies for chemoprevention in order to decrease the risk of developing cancer following exposure to total body irradiation (TBI) [4].

7.3 Adaptive Response

Space exploration exposes astronauts to the challenges of space radiation, posing potential risks to cellular systems. The adaptive response in space, as studied by researchers around the world, has the potential to contribute to the safety of astronauts during space travel. Mortazavi et al. in 2003 contributed to the study of adaptive response in space and its potential role in safeguarding astronauts during space expeditions. Their research focused on how a previous history of exposure to low-dose radiation can be used as an efficient method for decreasing the risk of radiation sickness and cancer after exposure to relatively high doses of radiation (e.g., large solar particle effects) through inducing adaptive response. These adaptive response studies may help choose astronauts for long-term space travel by identifying individuals with high adaptive responses to radiation.

Studies have shown that some humans living in very high natural radiation areas have acquired high adaptive responses to external radiation. These studies have been conducted in areas such as Guarapari, Brazil; Kerala, India; Ramsar, Iran; and Yangjiang, China, where people are exposed to high levels of natural radiation due to factors such as high levels of Ra-226 in the soil and rocks, radon-prone areas or monazite deposits [5–7]. Exposure to low doses of radiation can lead to activation of DNA repair and triggered apoptosis of damaged cells, which can make living organisms resistant to high doses of radiation. It has been suggested that measuring the adaptive response of potential crew members for long-term manned exploratory missions could help choose astronauts with the highest significant adaptive responses, which could reduce the risk of exposure to high-energy neutrons, protons, and high charge and energy particles during deep space missions [8, 9].

Some findings also suggest that radiofrequency-induced adaptive response can be used as an efficient method for decreasing the risk of infection after pre-exposure to radiation [10]. This is significant for space exploration, as the adaptive response may help mitigate the effects of radiation exposure and decrease the risk of infection, thus contributing to the overall safety and well-being of astronauts during long-term space missions.

Given the above considerations, individuals with significant adaptive responses may be better suited for long-term deep space missions [11, 12]. By measuring the adaptive response of potential crew members, it may be possible to select astronauts with high adaptive responses, thereby reducing their susceptibility to the detrimental effects of space radiation and minimizing the need for massive shielding. This could ultimately enhance the safety and well-being of astronauts during long-term space travel [13].

This section reviews the concept of radioadaptive response as a potential biological protective mechanism against the adverse effects of space radiation, considering its implications for the well-being of astronauts. Various studies exploring the adaptive response, its underlying mechanisms, and its potential as a countermeasure to space radiation exposure are discussed. Space radiation is a significant concern for long-duration space missions, and understanding the adaptive response becomes crucial for developing effective protective strategies.

Studies on cosmonauts involved in multiple space missions indicate lower-than-expected frequencies of chromosome aberrations, suggesting a potential adaptive response to repeated spaceflights [14]. p53-dependent adaptive responses in human cells exposed to space radiations are also explored [15]. Telomere length alterations as a potential biomarker for the adaptive response in space are discussed, highlighting NASA's findings on telomere elongation during space missions [16].

7.3.1 Time Dilation Vs. Telomere Elongation

As illustrated in Fig. 7.2, time dilation and telomere elongation are two fascinating phenomena observed in astronauts aboard the International Space Station (ISS). The ISS orbits the Earth at a speed of approximately 17,500 miles per hour, causing time to move more slowly for the astronauts compared to those on Earth. This effect, known as time dilation, is a key aspect of Einstein's theory of special relativity. An astronaut spending a year on the ISS would age about 0.014 seconds less than someone on the Earth, a small but scientifically significant confirmation of Einstein's theory.

Telomeres, on the other hand, are structures made from DNA sequences and proteins found at the ends of our chromosomes. They act like protective caps, preventing chromosomes from fraying or breaking. Each time a cell divides, telomeres shorten a bit. When they get too short, the cell can no longer divide and it dies, making telomeres a marker of cellular aging. Interestingly, during astronaut Scott Kelly's year in space, his telomeres unexpectedly lengthened by an average of 14.5%, an effect researchers on the Earth have been trying to achieve with an enzyme called telomerase.

It is worth noting that this elongation was temporary and the telomeres began shrinking back to preflight levels a few days after Scott's return to the Earth. While this observation is significant and shows adaptation to the harsh environment of space, it is not clear whether this can be interpreted as a marker of reverse aging. The changes observed in astronauts' telomeres and other genetic markers are part of ongoing research to understand the effects of long-term space travel on the human body. These studies will help guide future space missions and contribute to our understanding of human health in space.

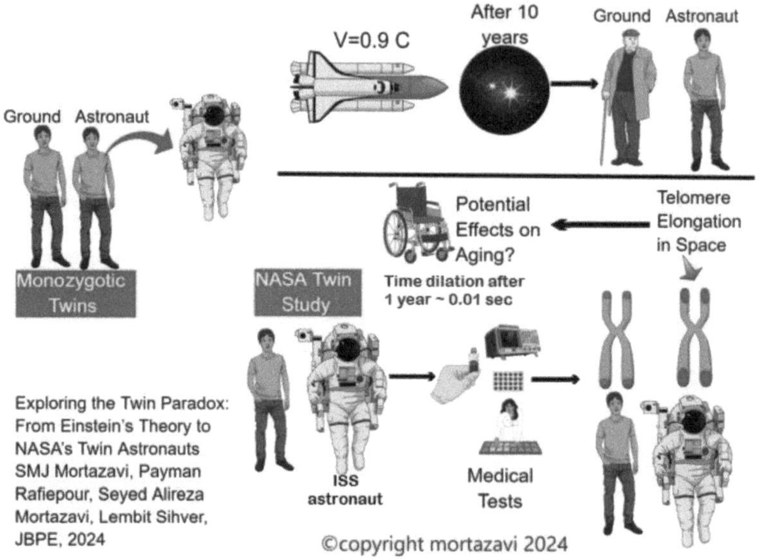

Figure 7.2 Time dilation on the ISS causes astronauts to age slightly slower than on the Earth, while telomeres unexpectedly lengthen during space missions but revert upon return, highlighting intriguing aspects of space travel on human biology.

Low-dose X-ray radiation has been investigated for its role in inducing an adaptive response, potentially serving as a countermeasure to galactic cosmic radiation exposure [17]. The involvement of oxidative stress and antioxidant pathways, including Akt and Nrf2 pathways, has been explored in the context of radiation-induced adaptive responses [18].

Studies on rat retinal cell cultures irradiated with γ-rays provide insights into the complexity of the adaptive response, involving DNA repair efficiency and the induction of antioxidant defenses [19]. Dose-response relationships for micronuclei induction by the combination radiation of α-particles and γ-rays in human lymphoblast cells are discussed, emphasizing the role of radiation-induced bystander effects [20]. The dependence of the adaptive response on radiation intensity is investigated, revealing that X-ray intensity plays a crucial role in inducing the adaptive response [21]. Additionally, adaptive responses in frogs chronically exposed to low doses of ionizing radiation in the environment are explored, suggesting stress-induced adaptation [22].

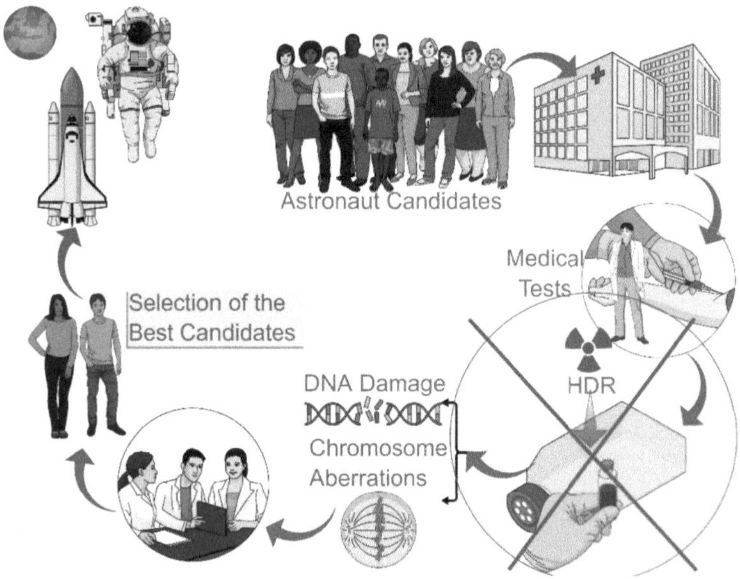

Figure 7.3 Clarifying misconceptions in candidate selection for space missions. It is a misconception that candidates with cells displaying maximum radiation resistance are necessarily the ones exhibiting the highest magnitude of adaptive response.

While there are misconceptions (Fig. 7.3), the proposed method, shown in Fig. 7.4, was developed by Mortazavi et al. They suggested that, before embarking on any long-term space mission, the adaptive response of all potential crew members should be assessed through routine cytogenetic tests. Subsequently, blood lymphocytes would be subjected to in vitro exposure, first to an adapting low dose and then to a challenging high dose. The magnitude of the observed adaptive response would be evaluated, and only those individuals demonstrating a high adaptive response should be selected for the mission. Throughout the mission, chronic exposure to elevated levels of space radiation is anticipated to significantly decrease radiation susceptibility. This strategy aims to better protect astronauts against unpredictable exposure to sudden and dramatic increases in flux resulting from solar particle events.

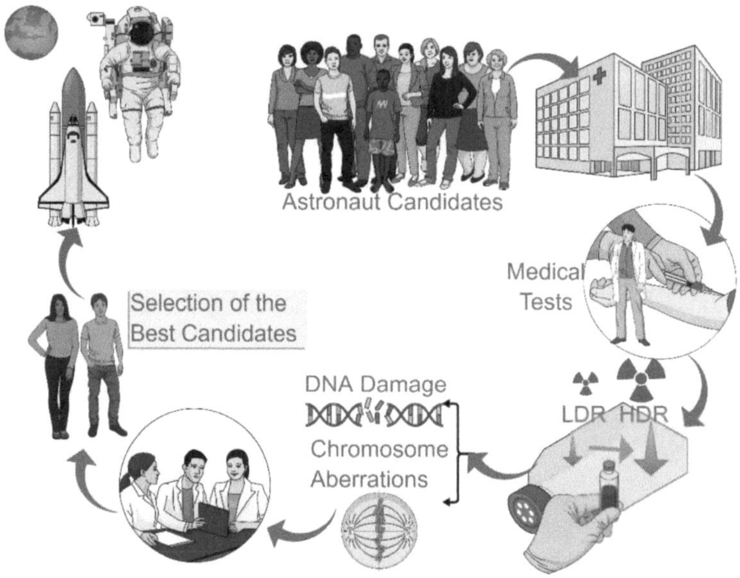

Figure 7.4 Optimal candidate selection method for deep space missions. Cultured lymphocytes of candidates undergo pre-exposure to low-dose radiation (LDR) followed by high-dose radiation (HDR) to determine the magnitude of adaptive response (MOAR). Candidates demonstrating the highest MOAR are considered ideal for missions to Mars and beyond.

As illustrated in Fig. 7.5, three adaptive response-based models have been proposed to address radiation risks during long-term manned space missions. In 2003, Mortazavi et al. introduced the adaptive response model, advocating its efficacy in reducing radiation risk. In 2018, Bevelacqua and Mortazavi refined this model, proposing routine cytogenetic tests for potential crew members. Selection would be based on a high adaptive response observed after exposing blood lymphocytes to both an adapting low dose and a challenging high dose, aiming to protect astronauts from chronic exposure and sudden increases in space radiation flux. NASA's model emphasizes understanding risks associated with the space environment, particularly the prevalence of protons. This awareness is crucial due to potential implications for adaptive response when cells encounter multiple instances of proton exposure. The Multiple Missions Model suggests that a first mission could serve as an adapting dose, and subsequent spaceflights may not significantly increase the risk of genetic abnormalities, indicating a possible natural defense mechanism or "radioadaptive response" against radiation exposure [8].

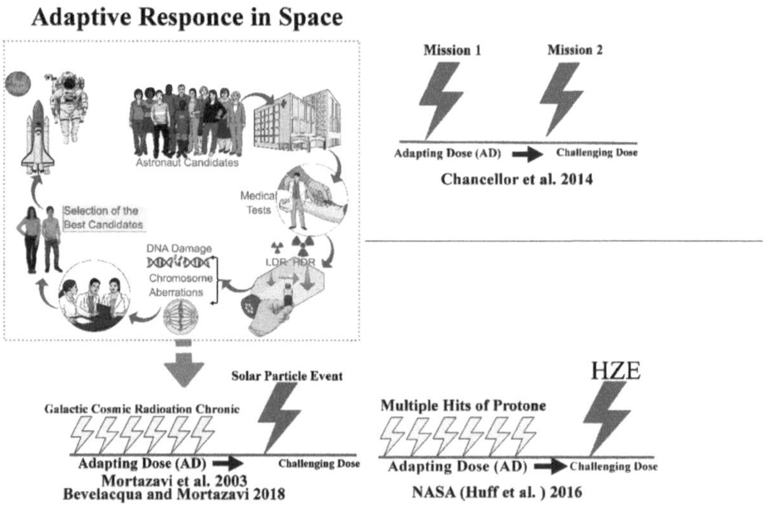

Figure 7.5 When astronauts demonstrating the highest MOAR are in space, the 3 models shown in the figure help astronauts resist high levels of radiation.

Despite promising findings, challenges in understanding the radioadaptive response, including variability in cellular models and irradiation protocols, should be taken into account. The potential relevance of adaptive response to space crew members is considered in light of specific exposure scenarios and dose rates [23]. Based on current knowledge of the radioadaptive response and its potential application in space radiation protection, further research is needed to better elucidate the underlying mechanisms and determine practical implications for astronaut well-being during space exploration.

7.4 Immunomodulation

Immunomodulation can help astronauts resist space radiation by addressing the immunosuppressive effects of microgravity and radiation exposure. Space travel, especially beyond lower Earth orbit, exposes astronauts to elevated radiation, which can lead to immune system dysregulation. Studies have shown that the microgravity environment during spaceflight severely impairs the immune system, making astronauts vulnerable to various diseases and increasing the risk of opportunistic viral infections [24–26]. The dysregulation of the immune system has been observed in both short-term and long-term space missions, leading to concerns about the ability of the immune system to respond and clear infections or pre-cancerous cells [25, 27]. Therefore, immunomodulation is crucial to counteract these effects and enhance the ability of the immune system to function effectively in the space environment.

The dysregulation of astronauts' immune systems can lead to the reactivation of latent viruses and persistent hypersensitivity reactions, which may increase specific clinical risks during deep space exploration missions. Bevelacqua et al. have reported that despite rigorous pre-mission screening and quarantine measures, it is possible for astronauts with a hidden or dormant SARS-CoV-2 infection to be sent to space. An astronaut with an inactive SARS-CoV-2 infection may pass all pre-launch medical tests without showing symptoms [28]. Then, during a long space mission such as a journey to Mars, the weakened immune system of these astronauts could allow the dormant infection to progress to a severe one, potentially impacting the success of the mission [29]. Factors such as microgravity, elevated space radiation, limited spacecraft size, close proximity of crew members, atmospheric composition, restricted exercise capability, and the potential for the virus to mutate and evolve during the mission all require further investigation [30].

Besides low doses of ionizing radiation, low levels of radiofrequency electromagnetic field (RF-EMF) may also have immunomodulatory effects. To investigate the effect of pre-exposure to RF-EMF on immune system modulation in a mouse model of hindlimb unloading (HU), the levels of T helper (Th)-mediated cytokines in the serum were measured using a multiplex cytometric bead assay in four different groups of mice, with 10 mice in each group [31]. The groups included mice subjected to simulated weightlessness (HU mice), mice exposed to RF-EMF-treated mice, HU mice that were pre-exposed to RF-EMF, and untreated control mice. The mice were exposed to 2450 MHz RF-EMF with a specific absorption rate (SAR) of 0.478 W/kg for 12 hours per day, over the course of three consecutive days. The impact of RF-EMF on HU mice showed that it can both increase IL-6 and decrease IL-9, indicating a potential regulatory effect on the changes induced by HU in these cytokines. This resulted in the eventual normalization of Th2 and Th9 levels, as well as the restoration of cytokine ratios in HU mice pre-exposed to RF-EMF [31].

While currently, we cannot provide specific details on how immunomodulation can directly help astronauts resist space radiation, based on existing knowledge, immunomodulation can potentially enhance the immune system's ability to recognize and eliminate damaged cells caused by radiation, as well as improve the body's defense against potential infections due to compromised immunity. This could be achieved through various strategies such as dietary supplements, pharmaceutical interventions, or targeted therapies to regulate immune responses and mitigate the adverse effects of space radiation on the immune system.

7.5 Physical Exercise

Space exploration poses unique challenges to the biological well-being of astronauts, including exposure to space radiation and the microgravity environment. This section explores the role of exercise as a countermeasure to mitigate the adverse effects of these challenges on the cardiovascular system, oxidative stress, bone health, immune function, and energy balance. The findings suggest that exercise, as a routine part of astronaut training, has potential protective effects on various physiological systems.

Studies indicate that exercise countermeasures play a crucial role in preserving cardiovascular health during space missions [32]. Although current exercise prescriptions on the International Space Station (ISS) help, there is a need for more effective strategies [33, 34]. Physical training has shown the potential to mitigate radiation damage from HZE ions [35]. Both exercise and spaceflight environmental factors contribute to oxidative stress. As will be discussed in the next section, prolonged high-intensity exercise can increase radical production, while moderate to low-intensity exercise may be beneficial in reducing oxidative stress induced by inactivity and hypoxia [36, 37]. However, caution is needed in applying these findings to deep-space environments [38].

Exercise, specifically running, shows promise in preventing bone mineral loss induced by radiation exposure in space [39]. Resistive exercise, when combined with pharmacological interventions, enhances the preservation of bone mass during prolonged spaceflights [40]. Exercise, incorporating both strength and aerobic training, helps counteract reductions in muscle strength and mass and has positive effects on the immune system [41]. However, the impact of exercise intensity on immune function needs consideration. Exercise affects energy balance during spaceflight, leading to a decrease in calorie consumption [42]. High-intensity interval training (HIIT) is proposed as a potential exercise countermeasure that minimizes energy expenditure while benefiting various physiological systems [43].

7.5.1 Disadvantages of Extreme Exercise in Space

Low-dose rate radiation exposure during space missions is examined in the context of oxidative stress. Studies reveal associations between radiation exposure and increased carotid intima-media thickness, vascular stiffness, inflammation, and insulin resistance [44–46]. The impact of space environment exposure on various tissues further emphasizes the multifaceted nature of oxidative stress induction. The complexities of conducting experiments in space, considering various influencing variables beyond radiation and microgravity, are discussed. The difficulty in isolating each factor's impact and the potential influence of spacecraft environmental conditions on results are acknowledged.

This section delves into the complexities of implementing exercise countermeasures in the microgravity environment of space, with a focus on potential complications arising from oxidative stress. While exercise is a critical component of maintaining astronaut health during space missions, the interplay between physical exertion and spaceflight environmental factors introduces challenges. The discussion draws attention to the amplified levels of oxidative stress caused by both physical exercise and spaceflight environmental factors, emphasizing the need for cautious optimization of exercise countermeasures. In their 2019 paper "Commentary: Introduction to the Frontiers Research Topic: Optimization of Exercise Countermeasures for Human Space Flight–Lessons From Terrestrial Physiology and Operational Considerations," Bevelacqua et al. have previously discussed that the positive or hormetic zone of exercise in space is much smaller for astronauts compared to their counterparts on the Earth due to key stressors such as space radiation and microgravity [47].

The effectiveness of exercise countermeasures for astronauts during space missions is explored, highlighting the need for optimization (Fig. 7.6). Despite the benefits of exercise in microgravity, the commentary by Bevelacqua et al. underscores a critical aspect overlooked by Scott et al. [48], the potential increase in oxidative stress due to physical exertion. The commentary by Bevelacqua et al. discusses the interconnection between physical exercise and Spaceflight Environmental Factors, illustrating how this combination significantly amplifies oxidative stress levels [49]. The potential transition from a beneficial to a harmful range of oxidative stress, especially when stressors coincide, is highlighted in Fig. 7.7, depicting the relationship.

The potential risks associated with high-duration and high-intensity exercise in space, leading to increased radical production and oxidative stress, are contrasted with the potential benefits of low-to-moderate-intensity exercise. The commentary by Bevelacqua and Mortazavi underscores the importance of exercising caution when evaluating tailored exercise levels for individual astronauts. Additionally, it highlights the potential interactions between physical exercise and other major stressors in space, particularly radiation. Their discussion prompts questions about the nature of combined exposure effects, urging a comprehensive assessment. In conclusion, it is emphasized that optimizing exercise countermeasures for astronauts should take into account the implications of oxidative stress. Their argument advocates for a nuanced approach, considering individual variability and potential interactions with other stressors in space.

In summary, exercise remains a critical component of astronaut training to address the challenges posed by space environments. While current exercise countermeasures on the ISS show promise, ongoing research is essential to refine exercise protocols and enhance their effectiveness in protecting astronauts' health during extended space missions.

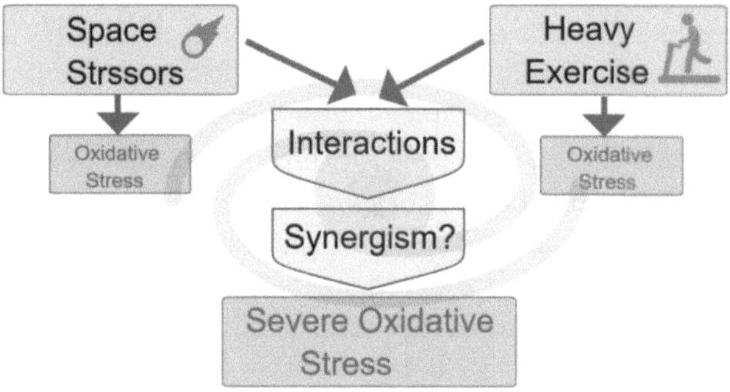

Figure 7.6 The effectiveness of exercise for astronauts in space is debated, particularly concerning the increase in oxidative stress. Current findings call for a nuanced approach to tailor exercise protocols, considering individual differences and interactions with environmental factors.

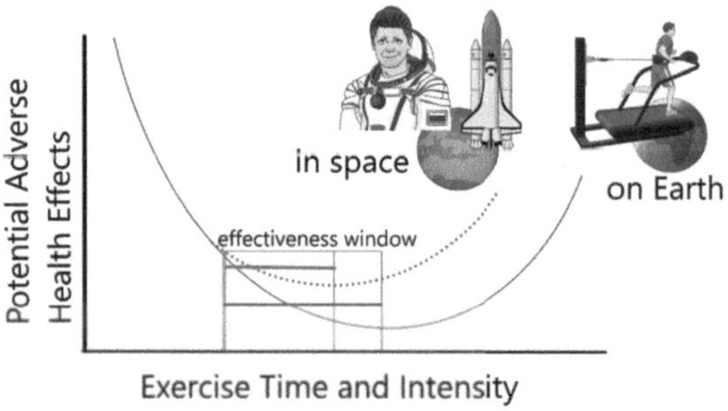

Figure 7.7 Considering the non-linear J-shaped relationship between the time and intensity of exercise and the potential of adverse health effects, we need a careful optimization of exercise intensity to prevent a transition from beneficial to harmful oxidative stress levels, especially when combined with other spaceflight stressors like radiation.

7.6 Mental Exercise

Since the inaugural life science space mission, notable physiological alterations have been recorded in various human systems including neurological, immunological, ophthalmological, and vestibular systems [50]. Despite advancements in space radiation research, significant challenges persist in accurately predicting and understanding human biological responses to radiation exposure [51]. In 1988, the National Council on Radiation Protection and Measurements (NCRP) issued Report No. 98: Guidance on Radiation Received in Space Activities [51, 52]. This document suggested limiting NASA astronauts to a lifetime radiation exposure that would not exceed a 3% risk of exposure-induced death (REID). This limit was underscored again in the 2015 NCRP Commentary No. 23: Radiation Protection for Space Activities: Supplement to Previous Recommendations, advocating for the continuation of the 3% REID limit for upcoming missions beyond LEO [51, 53].

Both radiation and microgravity have been shown to contribute to oxidative stress. Exposure to space radiation can induce oxidative stress in astronauts after extended spaceflight [54–58], while microgravity can cause oxidative stress and mitochondrial dysfunction [59–62]. Other stressors, such as fluid imbalances and limited resources, can also contribute to oxidative stress in astronauts [59, 63]. It is important to note that the effects of these stressors are interrelated and can compound each other through a synergistic effect, leading to a greater risk of oxidative stress and associated health problems [62]. Therefore, it is crucial to develop strategies to minimize oxidative stress and maintain the health of astronauts during long-duration spaceflight.

Oxidative stress is a great concern for astronauts due to reasons such as mitochondrial dysfunction, immunological stress, alterations in telomere length, arterial structure and function, and fluid balance. Studies have shown that astronauts could experience mitochondrial dysfunction due to oxidative stress [54]. Mitochondria are responsible for producing energy in cells, and when they are damaged, it can lead to a variety of health problems. Oxidative stress can also cause immunological stress in astronauts [54]. The count of white blood cells, particularly granulocytes, increases during spaceflight, while the count of lymphocytes decreases and the functions of immune cells are impaired. Despite the fact that the spaceflight environment raises the count of granulocytes in astronauts' blood, the molecular mechanisms responsible for this phenomenon are not yet understood [64]. This can weaken the immune system and make astronauts more susceptible to infections.

Telomeres are the protective caps on the ends of chromosomes that shorten as we age. Oxidative stress can cause telomeres to shorten more quickly, which can lead to premature aging and an increased risk of age-related diseases [54]. While in space, there is a temporary movement of fluid from the blood vessels to the cells, leading to a decrease in the overall volume of blood circulating in the body [65, 66]. At the same time, the return of blood to the heart and the amount of blood pumped with each heartbeat increase, which affects the activity of the autonomic nervous system and hormonal system [66, 67]. Long-duration spaceflight can cause changes in arterial structure and function due to oxidative stress [56]. This can increase the risk of atherosclerosis, which is the buildup of plaque in the arteries that can lead to heart disease [66].

Microgravity is another oxidative stress promoter that can cause fluid imbalances in the body [59]. This can lead to dehydration, electrolyte imbalances, and other health problems. The oxidative stress environment that is intensified during and after spaceflights, along with the mitochondrial dysfunction caused by radiation exposure, results in kidney damage at various levels [68]. This damage affects the integrity of both the tubules and glomeruli, as well as the function of micro- and macrovascular systems. Existing data indicates that the kidney experiences a significant oxidative stress assault during spaceflight, which is supported by studies detecting oxidation products in urine [68]. Increased oxidative stress is particularly obvious after spaceflight when damaged products are observed in the kidney [59].

The space environment is challenging, and resources are limited. Astronauts cannot easily access medical care or supplies, so preventing oxidative stress is crucial to maintaining their health and well-being [63]. In this context, oxidative stress is a great concern for astronauts due to its potential to cause a variety of health problems, including mitochondrial dysfunction, immunological stress, alterations in telomere length, changes in arterial structure and function, fluid imbalances, and increased oxidative stress.

Preventing oxidative stress is crucial to maintaining the health and well-being of astronauts during long-duration spaceflight [69].

In a study conducted by Im et al., it was discovered that Kouksundo, a traditional Korean mind-body practice with a long history, had a significant impact on reducing levels of oxidant markers in the body. This included reactive oxygen species, nitric oxide, and malondialdehyde [70]. Additionally, the practice increased levels of superoxide dismutase and decreased levels of catalase. These findings indicate that Kouksundo can effectively regulate oxidative stress and stress-related biomarkers. Overall, mind-body practices like Kouksundo have been shown to have positive effects on both mental and physical health [70]. Engaging in mental activities like playing chess may potentially contribute to the mitigation of oxidative stress through several mechanisms including increased brain function, neuroplasticity, stress reduction, social interaction, and cognitive reserve.

Mental activities, including playing chess, stimulate various regions of the brain associated with cognition, memory, and reasoning. This increased brain activity promotes the production of neurotrophic factors and neurotransmitters, which can help protect neurons against oxidative damage. Regular mental challenges provided by chess playing may enhance neuroplasticity, which is the brain's ability to adapt and reorganize itself. Neuroplasticity helps create new neural connections and strengthens existing ones, ultimately improving brain function and resilience against oxidative stress. Engaging in mentally stimulating activities like chess can help reduce stress levels. Chronic stress is known to increase oxidative stress in the body, and by reducing stress, chess playing may indirectly contribute to the mitigation of oxidative stress.

Chess is often played with others, promoting social engagement and interaction. Socializing has been linked to improved cognitive function and reduced oxidative stress. The positive social aspects of chess playing may contribute to overall well-being and indirectly impact oxidative stress levels. Regular mental activities, such as playing chess, have been associated with the development of cognitive reserve. Cognitive reserve refers to the brain's ability to adapt and function despite age-related changes or damage. This resilience may help mitigate the effects of oxidative stress on cognitive decline and neurodegenerative diseases. While these mechanisms provide potential explanations, further research is needed to establish a definitive link between engaging in mental activities like playing chess and the mitigation of oxidative stress.

7.7 Diet

Space exploration poses unique challenges to astronaut health, particularly in terms of exposure to space radiation and the effects of microgravity. This section reviews the role of diet and nutrition in providing biological protection against these challenges. The focus is on the radioprotective properties of indigenous Indian fruits, phytochemicals, and various nutritional countermeasures. The importance of adequate nutrition during long-duration spaceflight is emphasized, considering its impact on musculoskeletal, visual, cardiovascular, endocrine, and immune systems. The part also explores the potential of dietary supplements and functional foods to address the nutritional needs of astronauts, especially during extended missions where fresh food availability is limited.

Spaceflight induces alterations such as unintentional weight loss and dysregulation of the immune system [71]. Nutritional concerns include energy balance, micronutrient deficiencies, and fluid management. Various spaceflight-induced effects and proposed nutritional countermeasures are discussed, including oxidative stress, bone loss, muscle atrophy, microbiota alterations, and negative energy balance [72]. The manuscript [73] presents evidence that malnutrition or excess of certain nutrients can lead to biomolecule oxidation and cell injury.

The role of diet and nutrition in astronauts' health is investigated by many researchers. The radioprotective benefits of stone apple, mango, Indian gooseberry, black plum, and phalsa have been underscored. Mechanisms include free radical scavenging, antioxidant, anti-mutagenic, and anti-inflammatory effects. As well, scientific studies [74] reveal the effectiveness of fruits and phytochemicals in preventing radiation-induced ill effects. Clinical studies with Emblica officinalis and Punica granatum demonstrate mitigation of radiation-induced mucositis, dermatitis, and cystitis. Giardi et al. [75] highlight the protective effects of alpha-lipoic acid, vitamins A, B, and C, and β-carotene against radiation. The importance of maintaining micronutrient levels during spaceflight, especially selenium, is discussed. Long-duration spaceflight impacts astronaut health, with attention to musculoskeletal, visual, cardiovascular, endocrine, and immune systems [76].

A study conducted by Douglas et al. in 2021 evaluates the impact of galactic cosmic ray simulation on the nutritional content of foods, finding no significant differences immediately or one year after treatment [77]. Dried plum supplementation is effective in preventing bone loss caused by ionizing radiation [78]. The polyphenols in dried plum contribute to its antioxidant and anti-inflammatory properties. Pomegranate supplementation protects against radiation-induced depression-like behaviors. The synergistic effects of pomegranate polyphenols contribute to its antioxidant properties [79]. Dietary intake of omega-3 fatty acids mitigates systemic inflammation after radiation exposure [80]. In addition, omega-3 fatty acid supplementation may inhibit bone loss and enhance inflammation resolution during spaceflights [81–83]. Factors influencing individual responses to ionizing radiation, including age, sex, lifestyle, genetics, and diet, are explored [84]. Dietary antioxidants, such as vitamins and phenolic compounds, act as potent radioprotectors against oxidative stress [85]. Dietary agents have the potential to decrease oxidative damage induced by ionizing radiation [86]. However, Pisoschi and Pop have warned against the use of single dietary antioxidant agents that may alter other natural antioxidant defense mechanisms [87].

7.8 Gases

A study published in 2012 suggests a "systems biology" method that combines chemical and biological approaches to mitigate radiation exposure. The proposed method involves inhaling gas mixtures or consuming water with dissolved gases for these therapies [88]. It suggests using new medical gases for both scavenging radicals and signaling biological responses to exposure. The study of water radiochemistry, along with the impacts of gases like CO, H_2, NO, and H_2S on the body and the processes underlying radiation biology, suggests that this method could be advantageous for treating radiation exposure. Researchers also propose that it could be useful in managing other conditions linked to oxidative stress, including cardiovascular disease, cancer, chronic inflammatory diseases, hypertension, ischemia/reperfusion (IR) injury, acute respiratory distress syndrome, as well as Parkinson's and Alzheimer's diseases, cataracts, and aging.

7.9 Hibernation and Synthetic Torpor

Hibernation, a state of reduced metabolism, has long been considered a potential solution for extended space missions. Early proposals for hibernation in space exploration date back several decades, highlighting its relevance for missions exceeding 3–4 years [89]. This section explores the potential of hibernation and synthetic torpor as a biological strategy to protect astronauts from space radiation and microgravity during extended space missions. The investigation encompasses studies on various animal models, including ground squirrels, hamsters, mice, and zebrafish, with a focus on the molecular and physiological changes associated with hypothermia-induced radioprotection. The review also discusses the implications of reduced metabolic rates and altered gene expression patterns during hibernation and synthetic torpor, offering valuable insights for both space travel and cancer radiotherapy. The findings underscore the need for further experiments, especially in the context of long-term space missions, to understand and harness the radioprotective potential of hibernation and synthetic torpor.

Recently, synthetic torpor has emerged as a promising alternative, allowing the induction of a hypometabolic state in non-hibernating mammals [90]. Studies involving Wistar rats and hamsters have demonstrated increased radioresistance under hypothermic conditions, with a notable dose reduction factor (DRF) [91, 92]. Squirrels irradiated during hibernation exhibited higher survival rates, suggesting a complex relationship between temperature exposure and post-irradiation environments [93]. Prolonged hypothermia post-irradiation, however, resulted in intensified tissue damage upon returning to normal body temperature [94]. The role of thyroid administration and antithyroid substances in modulating radioresistance was explored, emphasizing the intricate interplay between metabolic rate and radiation lethality [95].

Given the active reduction in metabolic rate during torpor, the focus on mitochondrial activity has been pivotal. Torpor-induced reduction in oxygen consumption is suggested to halt tumor growth, as demonstrated in experiments with human tumors transplanted into hibernating hamsters [96]. Naturally occurring radioprotection in hibernating ground squirrels has been reported over a broad dose range [97]. The protective effects observed in hibernation are not solely attributed to the cessation of cell replication, warranting further investigation into the dynamics of DNA damage and repair pathways [98].

Poikilothermic animals provide valuable insights into the influence of low temperatures on radiation sensitivity. The "oxygen effect" and the role of tissue oxygenation in determining radiation sensitivity are discussed, with hypoxia leading to increased radioresistance [99–101]. The controversial role of conventional hypothermia, acting as both a protector and inhibitor of radiation damage repair, underscores the need for a comprehensive understanding of its long-term effects [90]. The hypothesis of hibernation as a radioprotective state is supported by experiments demonstrating decreased radiation-induced lethality during induced hypometabolic and hypothermic states [102]. A meta-analysis of rodent experiments further supports the notion that hibernation enhances radioresistance [89]. Melatonin, potentially acting as an antioxidant, is suggested to play a role in radioprotection during sleep [103].

Research on synthetic torpor reveals the downregulation of ATM and other DNA damage signaling genes, indicating a potential mechanism for increased radioresistance [90]. Pharmacological inhibition of ATM mimics the radioprotective effect observed in synthetic torpor, suggesting similarities between the two conditions [104]. Induced torpor in a zebrafish model demonstrates increased mitochondrial gene expression and decreased DNA damage compared to low-dose radiation exposure [105, 106]. A systems biology approach reveals the activation of pro-survival signaling and DNA repair pathways, emphasizing the potential for induced torpor as a radio-protectant [107].

In conclusion, the radioprotective mechanisms associated with hibernation and synthetic torpor remain incompletely understood and warrant further investigation. The implications of these findings extend beyond space travel to cancer radiotherapy, emphasizing the need for experiments exploring late effects at low radiation doses. Our review highlights the potential of induced torpor as a countermeasure for low-dose radiation exposure, providing valuable insights for future space exploration endeavors.

7.10 Probiotics

Probiotics have shown potential in protecting astronauts against the effects of space radiation and microgravity. Studies have demonstrated that probiotics, such as Lactobacillus and Bifidobacterium, exhibit improved tolerance to acid and bile, enhanced antimicrobial activity, and maintenance of adherence ability in simulated microgravity conditions [108]. Additionally, probiotics have been tested for stability during space travel, with promising results indicating their potential use in mitigating the health challenges faced by astronauts [109]. Furthermore, the use of probiotics has been associated with potential benefits such as maintaining the gut microbiome, preventing urinary tract infections, and modulating the immune system, which are particularly relevant for long-term space missions. While the research in this field is still in its early stages and largely based on animal models, the findings suggest that probiotics could be a valuable strategy to support astronaut health during space travel [110]. Moreover, given that astronauts are also exposed to galactic radiation, which can cause damage to the microbiome, the potential of probiotics to protect against such radiation-induced damage is an area of interest. Therefore, while further research is needed, the current evidence supports the prospective use of probiotics as a protective measure for astronauts in space.

7.11 Radioprotectors and Radiation Mitigators

Agents influencing the biological effects of ionizing radiation can be used in clinical radiotherapy and radiation protection including the protection of astronauts against space radiation. While radioprotectors are generally administered before exposure to radiation, radiomitigators can be used post-exposure to reduce the radiation damage. These compounds often act as antioxidants, boost DNA repair, possess anti-inflammatory properties, and prevent cell death. Radioprotectors and mitigators are of significant interest in protecting astronauts against the effects of space radiation. Space radiation, including galactic cosmic rays and solar particle events, poses a substantial risk to astronauts during long-duration missions beyond LEO. Radioprotectors are pharmacologic agents administered prior to radiation exposure to modulate the effects of radiation, while mitigators are given after exposure to reduce the symptoms or signs of radiation disease. Research has focused on the development of radioprotectors and mitigators to mitigate the biological consequences of space radiation, including the use of novel orally administered agents and immune system modulators [2]. While traditional radioprotectors such as amifostine are available, evidence suggests that radiation mitigators could play a crucial role in protecting astronauts during space missions. Ji et al. [111] have discussed the role of amifostine as a broad-spectrum radiation protection agent. The use of compound-based biological countermeasures to reduce the risk of space radiation-induced carcinogenesis, cardiovascular disease, and central nervous system deficiencies is considered imperative [112].

According to a report published on NASA's website, NASA has established a radiation limit of 600 mSv for astronauts throughout their careers [113]. However, upcoming missions beyond LEO, such as those to Mars, will subject the crew to at least double that amount of radiation. Sishc, the lead author of this report who is affiliated with Aegis Aerospace Houston, TX, believes that due to inherent limitations in spacecraft shielding against high-energy charged particles, alternative methods must be explored to reduce the overall risk of space radiation-induced health issues [113]. Recent successes in acute radiation syndrome and clinical radiotherapy have underscored the effectiveness of compound-based and biological interventions in alleviating the long-term health effects of space radiation exposure. They report that the Space Radiation Element of NASA has allocated funding for research into various compounds, including Avasopasem Manganese, CDDO-Me, Metformin, and γ-tocotrienol. These compounds have demonstrated efficacy in reducing the risks of carcinogenesis, central nervous system issues, and cardiovascular diseases [113]. We do believe that it is important to point out that natural mitigators like vitamin C, which can be used days after exposure to high levels of space radiation, are more effective than other countermeasures. Even after a significant solar particle event (SPE), there is sufficient time to utilize vitamin C [3]. This critical time window is essential for assessing any potential radiation countermeasure in space. Additionally, an ideal countermeasure should also be effective against the harmful effects of microgravity. We addressed this issue in our 2021 publication.

Mortazavi et al. have reported that vitamin C is a promising radiomitigator for astronauts due to its potential to reduce the detrimental effects of high levels of ionizing radiation, even when administered up to 24 hours after exposure. Their study, published in the Physica Medica, demonstrated that a single dose of vitamin C administered up to 24 hours after exposure to gamma radiation could potentially reduce the detrimental effects of high levels of ionizing radiation [114]. The survival rate in animals that received vitamin C, 1 hour, 12 hours, and 24 hours after irradiation were 55%, 60%, and 80%, respectively, and the viability of cells in animals that received vitamin C at those time points were 94.9%, 99.0%, and 100%, respectively. As for other natural radiation mitigators, a literature search does not provide specific information about any natural radiation mitigator that can be used 24 hours after radiation exposure. Therefore, vitamin C appears to be the most promising natural radiation mitigator that can be used 24 hours after radiation exposure [114]. Therefore, the development of effective radioprotectors and mitigators is essential to ensure the safety and health of astronauts during deep space missions [115, 116].

7.11.1 The Time Window of Effectiveness as a Challenge in Space Radiobiology

While radioprotectors are compounds that can protect against radiation injury when given prior to radiation exposure, mitigators can protect against radiation injury when given after exposure but before symptoms appear [117]. The duration of effectiveness of a mitigator after astronauts are exposed to a significant solar particle event (SPE) in space is a critical concern (Fig. 7.8). It is clear that an agent that remains effective for 24–48 hours or longer would be more beneficial compared to one that only works for a few hours after an

SPE [118]. Among the current candidates, amifostine is a protectant that reduces radiation damage to tissue if taken even minutes before radiation exposure. Neupogen® (filgrastim) is a medication that has effectively stimulated the production of white blood cells in cancer patients, reducing their susceptibility to infections. It is anticipated to provide similar benefits to patients with bone marrow damage caused by high doses of radiation. Neupogen can be taken after exposure to stimulate bone marrow for more rapid replenishment of white blood cells. Entolimod shows great promise in effectively reducing acute, potentially life-threatening radiation injuries in both small rodents and large NHPs. Given the thorough and detailed analyses conducted by the company, it is highly probable that humans suffering from similar radiation-related injuries would also see positive outcomes from entolimod treatment [119]. Entolimod can be given before or after exposure and has been shown to protect primates from damaging effects for up to 48 hours after exposure.

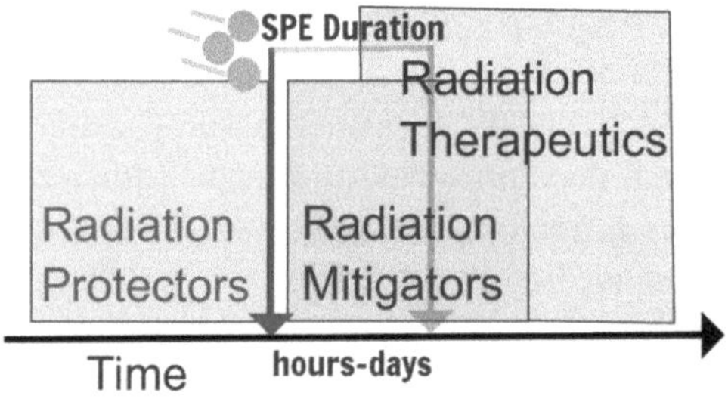

Figure 7.8 The length of time that a mitigator remains effective following exposure to a significant solar particle event (SPE) in space is of paramount importance. Agents that maintain efficacy for 24–48 hours or more are preferable to those that only offer a few hours of protection after an SPE.

Recilisib sodium (Ex-Rad), a synthetic chlorobenzyl sulfone derivative, is currently under investigation by Onconova Therapeutics and the US Department of Defense as a radiation shield. Research involving male mice has shown that administering Ex-Rad 24 hours and 15 minutes prior to radiation exposure resulted in an 88% survival rate. Both subcutaneous and oral administrations of Ex-Rad have been found to significantly enhance survival by mitigating radiation-induced damage, especially in protecting hematopoietic and gastrointestinal tissues. Mechanistic research indicates that Ex-

Rad promotes survival by activating the PI3-kinase/AKT pathway in cells exposed to radiation. Further studies have revealed that salidroside, a ROS scavenger, augments the radioprotective effects of Ex-Rad via a p53-dependent apoptotic pathway [120].

Romyelocel-L, also known as Plerixafor, is a medication employed to augment the quantity of stem cells in the bloodstream, a process referred to as stem cell mobilization. Specifically, it is utilized in conjunction with granulocyte colony-stimulating factor (G-CSF) to facilitate the mobilization of stem cells from the bone marrow into the bloodstream, where they can be gathered for transplantation. The mechanism of action of Romyelocel-L involves obstructing the interaction between the CXCR4 receptor on the surface of stem cells and its ligand, CXCL12, present in the bone marrow. Normally, this interaction confines stem cells within the bone marrow. However, by impeding it, Romyelocel-L enables the release of stem cells into the bloodstream. Administration of Romyelocel-L typically involves a single subcutaneous injection, and the subsequent collection of stem cells occurs through a process known as apheresis. This entails withdrawing blood from the body, separating the stem cells, and returning the remaining blood components to the body. Combining Romyelocel-L with G-CSF has demonstrated a significant increase in the yield of collected stem cells, thereby enhancing the success of stem cell transplantation. Romyelocel-L has the potential to mitigate damage even if administered 3–5 days after radiation exposure.

Amifostine shows potential as a radioprotector, but it has not been approved by the FDA for the treatment of acute radiation syndrome (ARS) due to the side effects associated with the necessary doses for radioprotection against ARS, as well as other significant clinical limitations [121]. However, it has been FDA-approved for specific uses, such as reducing the risk of kidney damage caused by cisplatin treatment in ovarian cancer patients and alleviating dry mouth in individuals undergoing radiotherapy for head and neck cancer [121].

We can conclude that radiation exposure is a significant threat to astronaut health during deep space missions, necessitating the development and refinement of various countermeasures. Beyond traditional passive and active shielding, essential strategies include genetic screening, radioprotectors, and radiomitigators. Additional measures like hibernation, immune system enhancement, and dietary adjustments are crucial for risk mitigation. Ongoing research is imperative to optimize these countermeasures, thereby ensuring astronaut safety and mission success.

References

1. Blue RS, Chancellor JC, Suresh R, Carnell LS, Reyes DP, Nowadly CD, et al. Challenges in clinical management of radiation-induced illnesses during exploration spaceflight. *Aerosp Med Hum Perform.* 2019; 90(11):966–77.
2. Montesinos CA, Khalid R, Cristea O, Greenberger JS, Epperly MW, Lemon JA, et al. Space radiation protection countermeasures in microgravity and planetary exploration. *Life* (Basel, Switzerland). 2021; 11(8).
3. Sihver L, Mortazavi SMJ. Biological protection in deep space missions. *J Biomed Phys Eng.* 2021; 11(6):663–74.
4. Montoro A, Obrador E, Mistry D, Forte GI, Bravatà V, Minafra L, et al. Radioprotectors, radiomitigators, and radiosensitizers. In: Baatout S, editor. *Radiobiology Textbook.* Cham: Springer International Publishing; 2023. p. 571–628.
5. Ghiassi-nejad M, Mortazavi SM, Cameron JR, Niroomand-rad A, Karam PA. Very high background radiation areas of Ramsar, Iran: preliminary biological studies. *Health Phys.* 2002; 82(1):87–93.
6. Hendry JH, Simon SL, Wojcik A, Sohrabi M, Burkart W, Cardis E, et al. Human exposure to high natural background radiation: what can it teach us about radiation risks? *J Radiol Prot.* 2009; 29(2a):A29–42.
7. Nishad S, Chauhan PK, Sowdhamini R, Ghosh A. Chronic exposure of humans to high level natural background radiation leads to robust expression of protective stress response proteins. *Scientific Reports.* 2021; 11(1):1777.
8. Bevelacqua JJ, Mortazavi SMJ. Commentary: human pathophysiological adaptations to the space environment. *Front Physiol.* 2017; 8:1116.
9. Mortazavi SM, Cameron JR, Niroomand-rad A. Adaptive response studies may help choose astronauts for long-term space travel. *Adv Space Res.* 2003; 31(6):1543–51.
10. Mortazavi SM, Motamedifar M, Namdari G, Taheri M, Mortazavi AR, Shokrpour N. Non-linear adaptive phenomena which decrease the risk of infection after pre-exposure to radiofrequency radiation. *Dose Response.* 2014; 12(2):233–45.

11. Mortazavi S, Cameron J, Niroomand-Rad A, editors. The life saving role of radioadaptive responses in long-term interplanetary space journeys. *International Congress Series*; 2005: Elsevier.

12. Mortazavi SM. Space radiobiology and the new era of induced radioresistance: should traditional concepts be moved to science history museums? *Technol Health Care*. 2013; 21(4):285–9.

13. Mortazavi SMJ, Said-Salman I, Mortazavi AR, El Khatib S, Sihver L. How the adaptation of the human microbiome to harsh space environment can determine the chances of success for a space mission to Mars and beyond. *Frontiers in Microbiology*. 2024; 14.

14. Durante M. Biomarkers of space radiation risk. *Radiation Research*. 2005; 164(4):467–73.

15. Takahashi A, Su X, Suzuki H, Omori K, Seki M, Hashizume T, et al. p53-dependent adaptive responses in human cells exposed to space radiations. *International Journal of Radiation Oncology* Biology* Physics*. 2010; 78(4):1171–6.

16. Welsh J, Keshavarz M. Is telomere length a biomarker of adaptive response in space? Curious findings from NASA and residents of high background radiation areas. *Journal of Biomedical Physics & Engineering*. 2019; 9(3):381.

17. Edwards S, Adams J, Tchernikov A, Edwards JG. Low-dose X-ray radiation induces an adaptive response: a potential countermeasure to galactic cosmic radiation exposure. *Experimental Physiology*. 2024.

18. Miura Y. Oxidative stress, radiation-adaptive responses, and aging. *Journal of Radiation Research*. 2004; 45(3):357–72.

19. Gaddini L, Bernardo A, Greco A, Campa A, Esposito G, Matteucci A. Adaptive response in rat retinal cell cultures irradiated with γ-rays. *International Journal of Molecular Sciences*. 2023; 24(3):1972.

20. Ren R, He M, Dong C, Xie Y, Ye S, Yuan D, et al. Dose response of micronuclei induced by combination radiation of α-particles and γ-rays in human lymphoblast cells. *Mutation Research/Fundamental and Molecular Mechanisms of Mutagenesis*. 2013; 741:51–6.

21. Shadley J, Wiencke J. Induction of the adaptive response by X-rays is dependent on radiation intensity. *International Journal of Radiation Biology*. 1989; 56(1):107–18.

22. Audette-Stuart M, Kim S, McMullin D, Festarini A, Yankovich T, Carr J, et al. Adaptive response in frogs chronically exposed to low doses of ionizing radiation in the environment. *Journal of Environmental Radioactivity*. 2011; 102(6):566–73.

23. Maalouf M, Durante M, Foray N. Biological effects of space radiation on human cells: history, advances and outcomes. *Journal of Radiation Research*. 2011; 52(2):126–46.

24. Lv H, Yang H, Jiang C, Shi J, Chen RA, Huang Q, et al. Microgravity and immune cells. *J R Soc Interface*. 2023; 20(199):20220869.

25. Crucian BE, Choukèr A, Simpson RJ, Mehta S, Marshall G, Smith SM, et al. Immune system dysregulation during spaceflight: potential countermeasures for deep space exploration missions. *Front Immunol.* 2018; 9:1437.

26. Bevelacqua JJ, Mortazavi SMJ. Commentary: immune system dysregulation during spaceflight: potential countermeasures for deep space exploration missions. *Front Immunol.* 2018; 9:2024.

27. Fisher R, Baselet B, Vermeesen R, Moreels M, Baatout S, Rahiman F, et al. Immunological changes during space travel: a ground-based evaluation of the impact of neutron dose rate on plasma cytokine levels in human whole blood cultures. *Frontiers in Physics*. 2020; 8.

28. Bevelacqua JJ, Mortazavi SA, Welsh JS, Mortazavi SMJ. How reactivation of SARS-CoV-2 in astronauts with dysregulated immune systems can negatively affect the odds of success in future space missions. *Journal of Biomedical Physics & Engineering*. 2023; 13(3):297–8.

29. Mortazavi S, Mortazavi S, Sihver L, editors. Can reactivation of SARS-CoV-2 decrease the chance of success of future deep space missions? *2021 IEEE Aerospace Conference* (50100); 2021, 6–13 March 2021.

30. Welsh JS, Bevelacqua JJ, Mozdarani H, Mortazavi SAR, Mortazavi SMJ. Why can COVID-19 fatality in space be significantly higher than on Earth? *Int-J-Radiat-Res.* 2020; 18(3):421–6.

31. Aghajari S, Mortazavi SMJ, Kalani M, Nematolahi S, Habibzadeh P, Farjadian S. The immunomodulatory effect of radiofrequency electromagnetic field on serum cytokine levels in A mouse model of hindlimb unloading. *Cell J.* 2021; 22(4):401–5.

32. Hughson RL, Helm A, Durante M. Heart in space: effect of the extraterrestrial environment on the cardiovascular system. *Nature Reviews Cardiology*. 2018; 15(3):167–80.

33. Hughson RL, Robertson AD, Arbeille P, Shoemaker JK, Rush JW, Fraser KS, et al. Increased postflight carotid artery stiffness and inflight insulin resistance resulting from 6-mo spaceflight in male and female astronauts. *American Journal of Physiology-Heart and Circulatory Physiology*. 2016; 310(5):H628–38.

34. Arbeille P, Provost R, Zuj K. Carotid and femoral artery intima-media thickness during 6 months of spaceflight. *Aerospace Medicine and Human Performance*. 2016; 87(5):449–53.

35. Kim DS, Weber T, Straube U, Hellweg CE, Nasser M, Green DA, et al. The potential of physical exercise to mitigate radiation damage—a systematic review. *Frontiers in Medicine*. 2021; 8:585483.

36. Powers SK, Radak Z, Ji LL. Exercise-induced oxidative stress: past, present and future. *The Journal of Physiology*. 2016; 594(18):5081–92.

37. Debevec T, Millet GP, Pialoux V. Hypoxia-induced oxidative stress modulation with physical activity. *Frontiers in Physiology*. 2017; 8:84.

38. Hellweg CE, Chishti AA, Diegeler S, Spitta LF, Henschenmacher B, Baumstark-Khan C. Molecular signaling in response to charged particle exposures and its importance in particle therapy. *International Journal of Particle Therapy*. 2018; 5(1):60–73.

39. Fukuda S, Iida H, Yan X. Preventive effects of running exercise on bones in heavy ion particle irradiated rats. *Journal of Radiation Research*. 2002; 43(Suppl):S233–S8.

40. Sibonga J, Matsumoto T, Jones J, Shapiro J, Lang T, Shackelford L, et al. Resistive exercise in astronauts on prolonged spaceflights provides partial protection against spaceflight-induced bone loss. *Bone*. 2019; 128:112037.

41. Crucian BE, Choukèr A, Simpson RJ, Mehta S, Marshall G, Smith SM, et al. Immune system dysregulation during spaceflight: potential countermeasures for deep space exploration missions. *Frontiers in Immunology*. 2018; 9:1437.

42. Zwart SR, Launius RD, Coen GK, Morgan JL, Charles JB, Smith SM. Body mass changes during long-duration spaceflight. *Aviation, Space, and Environmental Medicine*. 2014; 85(9):897–904.

43. Winding KM, Munch GW, Iepsen UW, Van Hall G, Pedersen BK, Mortensen SP. The effect on glycaemic control of low-volume high-intensity interval training versus endurance training in individuals with type 2 diabetes. *Diabetes, Obesity and Metabolism*. 2018; 20(5):1131–9.

44. Garrett-Bakelman FE, Darshi M, Green SJ, Gur RC, Lin L, Macias BR, et al. The NASA Twins Study: A multidimensional analysis of a year-long human spaceflight. 2019; 364(6436):eaau8650.

45. Arbeille P, Provost R, Zuj K, Carotid and femoral artery intima-media thickness during 6 months of spaceflight. 2016; 87(5):449–53.

46. Hughson RL, Robertson AD, Arbeille P, Shoemaker JK, Rush JW, Fraser KS, et al. Increased postflight carotid artery stiffness and inflight insulin resistance resulting from 6-mo spaceflight in male and female astronauts. 2016; 310(5):H628–38.
47. Bevelacqua JJ, Welsh J, Mortazavi S. Commentary: Introduction to the frontiers research topic: optimization of exercise countermeasures for human space flight–lessons from terrestrial physiology and operational considerations. *Frontiers in Physiology*. 2019; 10:915.
48. Scott JPR, Weber T, Green DA. Introduction to the frontiers research topic: optimization of exercise countermeasures for human space flight - lessons from terrestrial physiology and operational considerations. *Front Physiol*. 2019; 10:173.
49. Cooper C, Vollaard NB, Choueiri T, Wilson MJBst. Exercise, free radicals and oxidative stress. 2002; 30(2):280–5.
50. Mhatre SD, Iyer J, Puukila S, Paul AM, Tahimic CG, Rubinstein L, et al. Neuro-consequences of the spaceflight environment. 2022; 132:908–35.
51. Chancellor JC, Blue RS, Cengel KA, Auñón-Chancellor SM, Rubins KH, Katzgraber HG, et al. Limitations in predicting the space radiation health risk for exploration astronauts. 2018; 4(1):8.
52. NCRP. Guidance on radiation received in space activities: NCRP Report No. 98; 1988.
53. McKenna-Lawlor S, Bhardwaj A, Ferrari F, Kuznetsov N, Lal A, Li Y, et al. Feasibility study of astronaut standardized career dose limits in LEO and the outlook for BLEO. *Acta Astronautica*. 2014; 104(2):565–73.
54. Guan J, Wan XS, Zhou Z, Ware J, Donahue JJ, Biaglow JE, et al. Effects of dietary supplements on space radiation-induced oxidative stress in Sprague-Dawley rats. 2004; 162(5):572–9.
55. Kulkarni S, Gandhi D, Mehta PJ. Nutraceuticals for reducing radiation effects during space travel. *Handbook of Space Pharmaceuticals*. Springer; 2022. p. 915–33.
56. Li M, Gonon G, Buonanno M, Autsavapromporn N, de Toledo SM, Pain D, et al. Health risks of space exploration: targeted and nontargeted oxidative injury by high-charge and high-energy particles. 2014; 20(9):1501–23.
57. da Silveira WA, Fazelinia H, Rosenthal SB, Laiakis EC, Kim MS, Meydan C, et al. Comprehensive multi-omics analysis reveals mitochondrial stress as a central biological hub for spaceflight impact. 2020; 183(5):1185–201. e20.

58. Yu H, Gao Y, Zhou RJFiPH. Oxidative stress from exposure to the underground space environment. 2020; 8:579634.

59. Gómez X, Sanon S, Zambrano K, Asquel S, Bassantes M, Morales JE, et al. Key points for the development of antioxidant cocktails to prevent cellular stress and damage caused by reactive oxygen species (ROS) during manned space missions. 2021; 7(1):35.

60. Guarnieri S, Morabito C, Bevere M, Lanuti P, Mariggiò MAJOM, Longevity C. A protective strategy to counteract the oxidative stress induced by simulated microgravity on H9C2 cardiomyocytes. 2021; 2021:1–18.

61. Nguyen HP, Tran PH, Kim K-S, Yang S-GJnM. The effects of real and simulated microgravity on cellular mitochondrial function. 2021; 7(1):44.

62. Lee SM, Ribeiro L, Martin D, Smith SM, Zwart S, Laurie S, et al., editors. Defining the relationship between biomarkers of oxidative and inflammatory stress and the risk for atherosclerosis in astronauts during and after long-duration space flight (CARDIO OX). *Human Research Program Investigators' Workshop* (HRP IWS 2020); 2020.

63. Kumar A, Tahimic CG, Almeida EA, Globus RKJIJoMS. Spaceflight modulates the expression of key oxidative stress and cell cycle related genes in heart. 2021; 22(16):9088.

64. Paul AM, Mhatre SD, Cekanaviciute E, Schreurs A-S, Tahimic CG, Globus RK, et al. Neutrophil-to-lymphocyte ratio: a biomarker to monitor the immune status of astronauts. *Frontiers in Immunology.* 2020; 11:564950.

65. Iwase S, Nishimura N, Tanaka K, Mano T. Effects of microgravity on human physiology. *Beyond LEO-Human Health Issues for Deep Space Exploration.* 2020.

66. Patel SJIH, Vasculature. The effects of microgravity and space radiation on cardiovascular health: from low-Earth orbit and beyond. 2020; 30:100595.

67. Norsk P, Asmar A, Damgaard M, Christensen NJ. Fluid shifts, vasodilatation and ambulatory blood pressure reduction during long duration spaceflight. *The Journal of Physiology.* 2015; 593(3):573–84.

68. Pavlakou P, Dounousi E, Roumeliotis S, Eleftheriadis T, Liakopoulos VJIJoMS. Oxidative stress and the kidney in the space environment. 2018; 19(10):3176.

69. Steller JG, Alberts JR, Ronca AEJIjoms. Oxidative stress as cause, consequence, or biomarker of altered female reproduction and development in the space environment. 2018; 19(12):3729.

70. Im H-J, Kim Y-J, Kim H-G, Kim H-S, Son C-G. Kouksundo, a traditional Korean mind–body practice, regulates oxidative stress profiles and stress hormones. *Physiology & Behavior*. 2015; 141:9–16.
71. Chaloulakou S, Poulia KA, Karayiannis D. Physiological alterations in relation to space flight: the role of nutrition. *Nutrients*. 2022; 14(22):4896.
72. Gao R, Chilibeck PD. Nutritional interventions during bed rest and spaceflight: prevention of muscle mass and strength loss, bone resorption, glucose intolerance, and cardiovascular problems. *Nutrition Research*. 2020; 82:11–24.
73. Fang Y-Z, Yang S, Wu G. Free radicals, antioxidants, and nutrition. *Nutrition*. 2002;18(10): 872–9.
74. Raghu SV, Rao S, Kini V, Kudva AK, George T, Baliga MS. Fruits and their phytochemicals in mitigating the ill effects of ionizing radiation: review on the existing scientific evidence and way forward. *Food & Function*. 2023.
75. Giardi MT, Touloupakis E, Bertolotto D, Mascetti G. Preventive or potential therapeutic value of nutraceuticals against ionizing radiation-induced oxidative stress in exposed subjects and frequent fliers. *International Journal of Molecular Sciences*. 2013; 14(8):17168–92.
76. Montesinos CA, Khalid R, Cristea O, Greenberger JS, Epperly MW, Lemon JA, et al. Space radiation protection countermeasures in microgravity and planetary exploration. *Life*. 2021; 11(8):829.
77. Douglas GL, Cooper MR, Wu H, Gaza R, Guida P, Young M. Impact of galactic cosmic ray simulation on nutritional content of foods. *Life Sciences in Space Research*. 2021; 28:22–5.
78. Schreurs A-S, Shirazi-Fard Y, Shahnazari M, Alwood J, Truong T, Tahimic C, et al. Dried plum diet protects from bone loss caused by ionizing radiation. *Scientific Reports*. 2016; 6(1):1–11.
79. Dulcich MS, Hartman RE. Pomegranate supplementation improves affective and motor behavior in mice after radiation exposure. *Evidence-Based Complementary and Alternative Medicine*. 2013; 2013.
80. Little-Letsinger SE, Turner ND, Ford JR, Suva LJ, Bloomfield SA. Omega-3 fatty acid modulation of serum and osteocyte tumor necrosis factor-α in adult mice exposed to ionizing radiation. *Journal of Applied Physiology*. 2021; 130(3):627–39.
81. Chuong P, Wysoczynski M, Hellmann J. Do changes in innate immunity underlie the cardiovascular benefits of exercise? *Frontiers in Cardiovascular Medicine*. 2019; 6:70.

82. Zheng JJ, Pena Calderin E, Hill BG, Bhatnagar A, Hellmann J. Exercise promotes resolution of acute inflammation by catecholamine-mediated stimulation of Resolvin D1 biosynthesis. *Journal of Immunology* (Baltimore, Md: 1950). 2019; 203(11):3013–22.
83. Baba S, Smith T, Hellmann J, Bhatnagar A, Carter K, Vanhoover A, et al. Space flight diet-induced deficiency and response to gravity-free resistive exercise. *Nutrients.* 2020; 12(8).
84. Applegate KE, Rühm W, Wojcik A, Bourguignon M, Brenner A, Hamasaki K, et al. Individual response of humans to ionising radiation: governing factors and importance for radiological protection. *Radiat. Environ. Biophys.* 2020; 59(2):185–209.
85. Karabulutoglu M, Finnon R, Imaoka T, Friedl AA, Badie C. Influence of diet and metabolism on hematopoietic stem cells and leukemia development following ionizing radiation exposure. *Int J Radiat Biol.* 2019; 95(4):452–79.
86. Lemon JA, Boreham DR, Rollo CD. A complex dietary supplement extends longevity of mice. *The Journals of Gerontology Series A: Biological Sciences and Medical Sciences.* 2005; 60(3):275–9.
87. Pisoschi AM, Pop A. The role of antioxidants in the chemistry of oxidative stress: a review. *European Journal of Medicinal Chemistry.* 2015; 97:55–74.
88. Schoenfeld MP, Ansari RR, Nakao A, Wink D. A hypothesis on biological protection from space radiation through the use of new therapeutic gases as medical counter measures. *Medical Gas Research.* 2012; 2(1):8.
89. Cerri M, Tinganelli W, Negrini M, Helm A, Scifoni E, Tommasino F, et al. Hibernation for space travel: impact on radioprotection. *Life Sciences in Space Research.* 2016; 11:1–9.
90. Tinganelli W, Hitrec T, Romani F, Simoniello P, Squarcio F, Stanzani A, et al. Hibernation and radioprotection: gene expression in the liver and testicle of rats irradiated under synthetic torpor. *International Journal of Molecular Sciences.* 2019; 20(2):352.
91. Ignat'Ev D, Fialkovskaia L, Perepelkina N, Markevich L, Kraev I, Kolomiĭtseva I. The effect of hypothermia on the rat radioresistance. *Radiatsionnaia Biologiia, Radioecologiia.* 2006; 46(6):706–12.
92. Musacchia X. Hibernation, stress, intestinal functions, and catecholoamine turnover rate in hamsters and gerbils. 1973.
93. Barr R, Musacchia X. Postirradiation hibernation and radiation response of ground squirrels: telemetry surveillance. *Radiation Research.* 1972; 51(3):631–7.

94. Mraz L, Praslička M. Influence of hypothermia on the survival of mice after large doses of X-radiation. *Nature.* 1961; 189(4765):677–8.
95. Smith F, Grenan MM. Effect of hibernation upon survival time following whole-body irradiation in the marmot (Marmota monax). *Science.* 1951; 113(2946):686–8.
96. Lyman CP, Fawcett DW. The effect of hibernation on the growth of sarcoma in the hamster. *Cancer Research.* 1954; 14(1):25–8.
97. Musacchia X, Barr R. Survival of whole-body-irradiated hibernating and active ground squirrels: Citellus tridecemlineatus. *Radiation Research.* 1968; 33(2):348–56.
98. Baird BJ, Dickey JS, Nakamura AJ, Redon CE, Parekh P, Griko YV, et al. Hypothermia postpones DNA damage repair in irradiated cells and protects against cell killing. *Mutation Research/Fundamental and Molecular Mechanisms of Mutagenesis.* 2011; 711(1–2):142–9.
99. Gray LH, Conger AD, Ebert M, Hornsey S, Scott O. The concentration of oxygen dissolved in tissues at the time of irradiation as a factor in radiotherapy. *The British Journal of Radiology.* 1953; 26(312):638–48.
100. Conger AD. The effect of oxygen on the radiosensitivity of mammalian cells. *Radiology.* 1956; 66(1):63–9.
101. Hall EJ, Giaccia AJ. *Radiobiology for the Radiologist: Philadelphia*; 2006.
102. Ghosh S, Indracanti N, Joshi J, Ray J, Indraganti PK. Pharmacologically induced reversible hypometabolic state mitigates radiation induced lethality in mice. *Scientific Reports.* 2017; 7(1):14900.
103. Tordjman S, Chokron S, Delorme R, Charrier A, Bellissant E, Jaafari N, et al. Melatonin: pharmacology, functions and therapeutic benefits. *Current Neuropharmacology.* 2017; 15(3):434–43.
104. Heylmann D, Badura J, Becker H, Fahrer J, Kaina B. Sensitivity of CD3/CD28-stimulated versus non-stimulated lymphocytes to ionizing radiation and genotoxic anticancer drugs: key role of ATM in the differential radiation response. *Cell Death & Disease.* 2018; 9(11):1053.
105. Cahill T, da Silveira WA, Renaud L, Williamson T, Wang H, Chung D, et al. Induced torpor as a countermeasure for low dose radiation exposure in a zebrafish model. *Cells.* 2021; 10(4):906.
106. Cahill T, Chan S, Overton IM, Hardiman G. Transcriptome profiling reveals enhanced mitochondrial activity as a cold adaptive strategy to hypothermia in zebrafish muscle. *Cells.* 2023; 12(10):1366.
107. Cahill T, da Silveira WA, Renaud L, Wang H, Williamson T, Chung D, et al. Investigating the effects of chronic low-dose radiation exposure in the liver of a hypothermic zebrafish model. *Scientific Reports.* 2023; 13(1):918.

108. Bharindwal S, Goswami N, Jha P, Pandey S, Jobby R. Prospective use of probiotics to maintain astronaut health during spaceflight. *Life* (Basel, Switzerland). 2023; 13(3).

109. Siddiqui R, Qaisar R, Goswami N, Khan NA, Elmoselhi A. Effect of microgravity environment on gut microbiome and angiogenesis. *Life* (Basel). 2021; 11(10).

110. Turroni S, Magnani M, KC P, Lesnik P, Vidal H, Heer M. Gut microbiome and space travelers' health: state of the art and possible pro/prebiotic strategies for long-term space missions. 2020; 11.

111. Ji L, Cui P, Zhou S, Qiu L, Huang H, Wang C, et al. Advances of amifostine in radiation protection: administration and delivery. *Molecular Pharmaceutics*. 2023; 20(11):5383–95.

112. Sishc BJ, Zawaski J, Saha J, Carnell LS, Fabre KM, Elgart SR. The need for biological countermeasures to mitigate the risk of space radiation-induced carcinogenesis, cardiovascular disease, and central nervous system deficiencies. *Life Sciences in Space Research*. 2022; 35:4–8.

113. Sishc BJ, Zawaski JA, Saha J, Nelson GG, Elgart SR, editors. Biological space radiation countermeasures to enable long duration exploration missions. *International Congress on Radiation Research (ICRR) 2023 Annual Meeting*; 2023.

114. Mortazavi S, Sharif-Zadeh S, Mozdarani H, Foadi M, Haghani M, Sabet E. Future role of vitamin C in radiation mitigation and its possible applications in manned deep space missions: survival study and the measurement of cell viability. *Physica Medica: European Journal of Medical Physics*. 2014; 30:e97.

115. Mortazavi SM, Rahimi S, Mosleh-Shirazi MA, Arjomandi M, Soleimani A, Koohi Hossein-Abadi O, et al. A comparative study on the life-saving radioprotective effects of vitamins A, E, C and over-the-counter multivitamins. *J Biomed Phys Eng*. 2015; 5(2):59–66.

116. Mortazavi SMJ, Foadi M, Mozdarani H, Haghani M, Mosleh-Shirazi MA, Abolghasemi P, et al. Future role of vitamin C in radiation mitigation and its possible applications in manned deep space missions: survival study and the measurement of cell viability. *International Journal of Radiation Research*. 2015; 13(1):55–60.

117. Rosen EM, Day R, Singh VK. New approaches to radiation protection. *Frontiers in Oncology*. 2014; 4:381.

118. Mortazavi SMJ, Foadi M, Mozdarani H, Haghani M, Mosleh-Shirazi MA, Abolghasemi P, et al. Future role of vitamin C in radiation mitigation and its possible applications in manned deep space missions: survival

study and the measurement of cell viability. *International Journal of Radiation Research*. 2015; 13(1):55–60.

119. Singh VK, Seed TM. Entolimod as a radiation countermeasure for acute radiation syndrome. *Drug Discovery Today*. 2021; 26(1):17–30.
120. Obrador E, Salvador R, Villaescusa JI, Soriano JM, Estrela JM, Montoro A. Radioprotection and radiomitigation: from the bench to clinical practice. *Biomedicines*. 2020; 8(11).
121. Singh VK, Seed TM. The efficacy and safety of amifostine for the acute radiation syndrome. *Expert Opinion on Drug Safety*. 2019; 18(11):1077–90.

Chapter 8

Social Attitudes to Ionizing Radiation

Wade Allison
Keble College, University of Oxford, UK
wade.allison@physics.ox.ac.uk

Like fire, ionizing radiation can be dangerous to life, but a detailed scientific understanding should underpin its regulation and the public should be given simple guidance for their safety. For 45 years after the discovery of X-rays in 1895 and nuclear radiation in the following years, ionizing radiation and its technology were trusted by society as a source of welcome benefits to health. However, due to political and other reasons that confidence was lost. That trust should be rebuilt to facilitate a viable social and economic future for the world in a changing climate.

Ionizing radiation impacts life on three distinct scales: (a) the physical response, (b) the biological reaction, and (c) the attitude of society. Each has its time frame and logic. Providing a scientific culture that acknowledges and recognizes how these fit together presents a significant but soluble problem, even though it will take some decades for its benefits to permeate public opinion.

Radioactivity in Life Sciences
Edited by Maria Letizia Terranova

ISBN 978-981-5129-67-0 (Hardcover), 978-1-003-63654-0 (eBook)
www.jennystanford.com

8.1 Introduction

Society is particularly wary of unseen dangers, such as poisoned food and infection by a virus or bacterium. So too, exposure to ionizing radiation cannot be felt, even at dangerous levels. Animals, birds, and fish are not aware of it either. Even humans only learn of its presence from those who have instruments able to detect it. As a result, they worry about it, uncertain whether they can trust what they are told and cannot themselves confirm. To be effective public policy should be built on a proper scientific description of the risks involved and include an educational strategy to share experience and confidence with the population at large.

The initial effect of exposure to ionizing radiation usually occurs within seconds. This is the stage determined by physical science. The second stage is the biological response to this attack, which takes place over an interval of hours and days. The third phase is exclusive to humans and may take years or even decades. It concerns the personal reaction to being informed of exposure to radiation, and thence the collective social and economic consequences. Since there is no direct sensory awareness, the social reaction relies on confidence in science and authorities. A lack of such confidence can lead to instability, even panic.

Appropriate safety and public policy rely on a balanced appreciation of all three responses—the physical reaction, the biological response, and the personal and social consequences. In the following each of these is discussed, in turn, several scientific and historical misunderstandings are clarified in the process.

8.2 The Physical Response

8.2.1 Why Ionizing Radiation Is Different

The year 1905 was extraordinary, even for Albert Einstein. He published his "Special Relativity Theory," his account of "Brownian Motion," and his explanation of the "Photoelectric Effect," all in the same year. Any of these would have deserved the Nobel Prize. In fact, it was for the latter, he received it in 1920. In it, he used the Quantum Theory, that Max Planck had hypothesized in 1900 to account for the spectrum of black body radiation. Einstein explained how, when ionizing radiation is absorbed by any material, it is not absorbed uniformly like most radiation, but as a series of discrete "collisions" in which a photon, a quantum of radiation as suggested by Planck, knocks out an electron from an atom of a target material. This instant emission of individual ionization electrons is quite different from the gradual heating that accompanies the absorption of non-ionizing radiation.

The problem that Einstein addressed in 1905 was the absorption of ultraviolet light by a simple metal surface. In that case, there is a simple threshold in the photon energy spectrum for the photoelectric emission of a free electron. Extended to a general material, energy absorption is similarly quantized in terms of photon absorption, which may excite a resonant state or induce a non-thermal molecular change.

How far ionizing radiation penetrates an absorbing material is described as the rate at which its intensity falls with distance. For electromagnetic radiation, this attenuation comes from the probability of a "collision" that falls as the intensity falls. As a result, the penetration distribution, $R(x)$, falls off exponentially, with a mean range λ_{abs}, thus:

$$R(x) = R(0)\exp(-x/\lambda_{abs}).$$

In addition, there may be secondary radiation emitted in the absorption process, each with its energy, direction, and type, such as the scattered photon and recoil electron emitted in the Compton process.

8.2.2 Radiation and Energy

Radiation is energy in motion. As such, it has many manifestations including sound, water waves, radio, microwaves, and light. Generally, the energy of these is rather harmless unless the intensity is raised. When that happens, they heat materials that absorb them, and the increased temperature can be felt. For example, the safety of a clinical ultrasound scan is assessed by comparing its heating with the resting metabolic rate of about 1 watt per kg. Tissue readily copes with such heat dissipation by circulation and perspiration. The same heating criterion is considered for the safety of radiofrequency (RF) absorption in a magnetic resonance imaging (MRI) scan [1].

However, the effect of ionizing radiation is quite different, and so too is its safety scenario. Let us first explain the meaning of energy in the context of ionizing radiation. We begin by considering radiation in the form of electromagnetic energy with its spectrum stretching from radio waves to X-rays and gamma rays.[1] Later, we extend the discussion of ionizing radiation to include high-velocity electrons (beta radiation), helium nuclei (alpha radiation), and protons (Fig. 8.1).

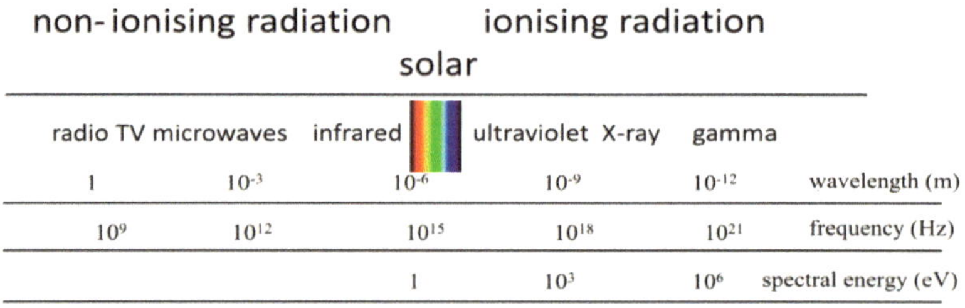

Figure 8.1 The electromagnetic spectrum.

The *energy* of radiation, as a measure, has two distinct meanings.

- There is the energy in joules (J), the integrated intensity delivered and absorbed to a mass of material over a period of time. We refer to this energy per kg of exposed tissue or material as the *radiation dose*, measured in joules per kg or gray (1 Gy = 1 J kg^{-1}). A given dose may be received slowly at a low dose rate or rapidly at a high dose rate. Both the dose and its rate are important. Significantly, the dose may be *acute*, i.e., one shot integrated over time and measured in Gy. Alternatively, the dose may be *chronic*, delivered continuously for an indefinite period at a certain dose rate, expressed in Gy per hour or month, for example. Between the two extremes, a specific dose in Gy may delivered over a protracted time at a certain dose rate.
- However, usually, the *energy* of ionizing radiation refers, not to its intensity or dose, but to its characteristic *spectral energy*, its 'color' in fact, as described by its wavelength in meters, λ, or its frequency in s^{-1}, ν, with $\lambda\nu = c$, where c is the velocity

[1]There is no real difference between X-rays and gamma rays except their energy, whether they come from nuclear decay or atoms and accelerators.

of light. The spectral energy affects the safety of a dose of ionizing radiation because it is quantized. The energy of a quantum is $h\nu$ joules where h is Planck's constant, 6.26×10^{-34} joule seconds. This is often expressed in electron volts (eV) by dividing by the electron charge 1.6×10^{-19} coulombs.

In addition to the absorbed dose per kg in Gy, measurements of ionizing radiation describe the rate of emission of particles or quanta by a source. One becquerel (Bq) is an emission of one per second. The relation between the activity of a source in Bq and the dose received by an absorber in Gy depends on how much of the radiation is absorbed by the material of interest, mass M, rather than going elsewhere. If all of the radiation is absorbed and the spectral energy of the radiation is E, then in an exposure time T, the dose D in Gy is related to the activity A in Bq by:

$$D = A \times E \times T / M.$$

From a safety perspective, the important quantities are the dose D and dose rate D/T, not A.

How does the safety of ionizing radiation compare with the safety of ultrasound or the RF radiation absorbed in an MRI scan? A preliminary answer can be given by reference to a dose rate that is fatal to cancer cells in a course of radiotherapy treatment. Such an absorbed dose rate is about 2 Gy per day, given for a month or more. That rate of energy absorption is $2/(24 \times 3600)$ or 20 microwatts per kg—some 50,000 times smaller than a level that is safe for clinical ultrasound or MRI. So, it is no surprise that ionizing radiation cannot be felt. But it also raises the obvious question—what makes ionizing radiation so much more dangerous than other types of radiation?

Ionizing radiation acts at the microscopic level, i.e., on materials through their atomic and molecular structure. In particular, it delivers energy to electrons, simply because, being the lightest particles in matter, they are most easily accelerated by the electromagnetic fields inherent in the radiation. Atomic nuclei are 2000 to 500,000 times heavier than an electron, as well as being 100,000 times smaller than atoms. Consequently, nuclei are not normally involved in absorption—they only have a role as possible *sources* of ionizing radiation. This observation has crucial practical consequences for radiological safety that should be widely appreciated—but seldom are. "*Radiation does not make materials radioactive*"[2] and thence "*You cannot catch radioactivity—it is not contagious like fire or a virus.*"[3]

8.2.3 Linearity in Physical Absorption

These phenomena, whether absorption or emission of ionizing radiation is a non-thermal statistical process determined by quantum mechanics. It is linear, a fundamental feature in much of mathematical physics. This means that the absorption or emission of each quantum of radiation, whether an electron or a photon, is independent of the others. It follows that the damage caused by the absorption of many electrons or photons just accumulates in proportion. The intensity of the radiation simply determines the number of independent "collisions" without any threshold in intensity or dose absorbed. This holds true whether the absorbing material is alive or dead.

This property of the physical stage of radiation absorption is central to the so-called linear no-threshold (LNT) model of radiological protection. It implies that the resulting damage adds up in the same way, regardless of whether the radiation dose is delivered spread out in time, or even received by different people. From a regulatory point of view, this is rather convenient. The *effective dose* is calculated by simply adding up all the doses for everyone in the population whether small or large. It is supposed that a simple coefficient should provide a realistic estimate of the damage caused, for instance, the number of cancers or the number of radiation-induced deaths. However, this LNT model argument is flawed because it ignores the biological response. It might be appropriate for a dead absorber, but not a live one, as explained later.

It might be supposed that to describe the relationship between cause and effect more effectively, a different function than a straight line through the origin might be used—or a quadratic curve. But this is to misunderstand linearity. It is not a choice of mathematical

[2]Except in the case of neutron radiation, it is very rare in the environment.

[3]Awful reports can be found in the media following a nuclear accident in which people, thought to have been irradiated, are turned away from hospitals and places of refuge and treated by others as contaminated. Those in authority are never told that this is not just inhumane but simply unjustified, scientifically.

simplicity, but of causality—that each element of absorbed radiation causes an element of radiation damage, and this relationship is unique.

8.2.4 Sources and Types of Ionizing Radiation

Electromagnetic radiation may be produced by de-celebrating electrons, effectively the inverse of the absorption process. This is called Bremsstrahlung or braking radiation. The brake is provided by the electric field of the highly charged nucleus of a high *Z* atom, such as Tungsten. Such radiation was named X-rays by Rőntgen, who discovered the phenomenon in 1895. Alternatively, ionizing radiation can be emitted in the electromagnetic decay of an excited nucleus, such as Technetium-99m.

The properties of the radiation must not depend on where the radiation comes from, only on its spectral energy and type, for instance, alpha, beta, or gamma. In the case of alpha and gamma radiation, the energy is directly related to the mass difference[4] between the initial and final nucleus multiplied by c^2. For beta-radioactive decay, this available energy has to be shared between the electron (or positron) and an outgoing unseen neutrino. As a result, the energy of a beta electron may be much less than the full energy of the decay process and has a broad spread. For instance, in the decay of tritium, the half-life is 12.32 years and the maximum energy is 18.6 keV, with a mean of 5.7 keV, the rest being taken by the neutrino. This energy is exceptionally low among beta decays and is relevant to a significant public incident.

In 2023, Japan had accumulated 1.19 million tons of cooling water from the Fukushima accident in 2011 and wanted to discharge it into the Pacific Ocean. The IAEA declared this to be safe after the water had been chemically filtered of all elements except for 16 grams of tritium. The water was to be diluted before release, but what radiation dose would be given by drinking a liter undiluted? Each decay electron carries an average energy of (5.7×10^3) $(1.602 \times 10^{-19}) = 0.91 \times 10^{-15}$ joules. The 16 g of tritium comprised 32×10^{23}

[4]The relation between energy release and the mass difference is universal for all energy, whether nuclear, chemical, or dropping from a height. In nuclear phenomena, the mass differences may be larger, but the relationship $E = mc^2$ is not peculiar to nuclear energy as popularly supposed.

atoms. The mean life is 12.32 / 0.693 (31 × 10^6) = 55 × 10^7 seconds. So, the total decay rate is 0.58 × 10^{16} Bq in the 1.19 × 10^9 kg of water. A glass of 100 ml of water would contain an activity of 0.48 × 10^6 Bq. Tritiated water behaves like ordinary water. The average time of any drunk water that is gradually lost from a body is 15 days. In that time, a total of 0.62 × 10^{12} decays from the glass of water occur in the body, each with 0.91 × 10^{-15} joules of energy. For a person of 70 kg that is a dose of (0.62 × 10^{12}) (0.91 × 10^{-15}/ 70) = 8 × 10^{-6} Gy over the 15 days. That is less than 1/1000 of the dose of a CT scan at 10^{-2} Gy. In other words, the radiation dose from one CT scan is equivalent to drinking 100 liters, i.e., a tenth of a ton, of undiluted cooling water from Fukushima Daiichi, all within 15 days! Evidently, the real problem is trust, not radiation at all.

Charged particle radiation is a form of ionizing radiation that includes high-speed electrons, protons, and alpha particles (nuclei of Helium-4). Being charged, their electromagnetic fields collide with atomic electrons in the absorbing medium transferring energy to them. Importantly, these collisions are atomic, not nuclear. So, they have high cross sections but modest transfers of energy. As a result, incident electrons, protons, and alpha particles lose energy with distance gradually. The rate is proportional to z^2/β^2 where the charge is ze and the speed βc. This factor is called the linear energy transfer (LET), which is effectively unity for beta rays. The collision of a high-energy electron with an atom or molecule involves quantum probabilities, which are closely related to those for a photon. So, both are described as low LET radiation. The difference is that an electron scatters and gradually loses energy in collisions until it stops. So, it has a relatively well-defined range, unlike that of a photon which is distributed exponentially. Alpha radiation has a high LET factor because its z is 2 and its mass is 8000 times that of an electron. Consequently, for a given energy, its speed βc is small and its rate of energy loss is very high. Significantly, the damage caused per unit dose in Gy is found to be higher by an extra factor of about 20. This factor, the relative biological effectiveness (RBE), is an empirical ad hoc feature that is appended to the LNT model without explanation or precise value. However, it is a likely consequence of the extra localized concentration of energy deposition as it affects the biological repair mechanisms to be discussed in the next section. With its high LET alpha radiation has a short range and is stopped by a sheet of paper or a layer of skin. If a source of alpha radiation is ingested, none of its energy escapes the body. That was the fate of the unfortunate Alexander Litvinenko, who was murdered by the Russian Secret Service with a dose of between 1000 and 3000 MBq of Polonium-210 [2].

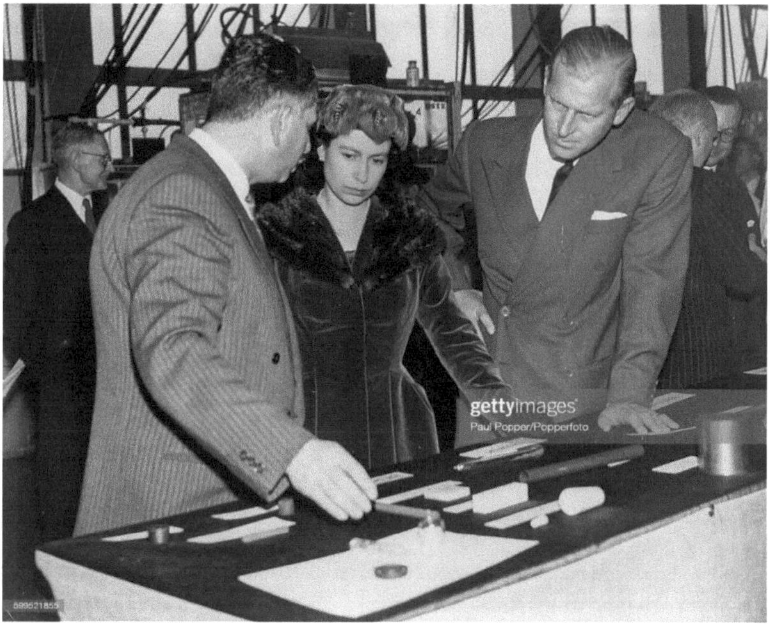

Figure 8.2 Queen Elizabeth at Harwell in 1957.

That contrasts with the effect of an external alpha source, which is harmless, as the following true story illustrates [3]. On a visit to Harwell in 1957, the young Queen Elizabeth was given a bag of Pu-239 to hold and feel its warmth—Plutonium, the element that the media understands as the most dangerous on the Earth (Fig. 8.2). Its decay emits an alpha particle of energy 5.245 MeV with a range too short to get through the simple bag. So, no radiation reached the Queen. The Pu-239 half-life of 24,200 years means the activity is 2.33 × 10^{12} decays per second per kg. Each alpha particle carries 0.84 × 10^{-12} joules. The product of these is 1.96 watts per kg, a little above the resting metabolic rate of normal tissue. No doubt, the bag did feel pleasantly warm to the Queen when she felt it. Her health was not affected and she lived for another 65 years. The media would not be inclined to believe this story, but the simple calculation confirms how warm the bag would have felt.

Proton radiation is produced, not by radioactive decay, but by accelerating protons obtained by ionizing hydrogen. When it enters tissue or any other material, it loses energy slowly at first and progressively more intensively as its speed βc falls and its LET rises. Near where it stops, it delivers most of its energy, the so-called "Bragg peak." This has the most important clinical applications in modern proton cancer radiotherapy where the energy delivered can be concentrated at the depth just where the tumor is located. In addition, the beam of protons can be steered and focused magnetically. None of these features is possible with X-rays and gamma rays. Problem is that the protons have to be accelerated to sufficient energy, about 250 MeV, for them to penetrate deep enough. The availability of suitable accelerators has limited the introduction of such therapy.

8.3 The Biological Response

8.3.1 Cause, Effect, and Feedback

Tissue has a composite structure of cells and fluids so it matters which atoms, molecules, and cells are damaged in the collision process. The immediate strike generates secondary energetic products that themselves create further damage. These include free electrons and reactive oxidant species (ROS). Since more than 50% of the tissue is water, these ROS include excited fragments like OH. The absorption of ionizing radiation generates many such oxidizing agents, similar to those from random chemical oxidation that arise during metabolic processes, resting or enhanced by exercise. Damage to the critical DNA molecules in the nucleus of a cell may be caused by the initial strike of radiation, its secondary ROS agents, or by oxidation unrelated to radiation.

The initial physical damage to biological tissue from a dose of ionizing radiation may be linear, but what happens subsequently distinguishes living tissue from inanimate material. If it is passive like a radiation monitor or film badge, it would accumulate a record of all damage received, but significantly it does not. After a time, a radiation monitor record is no longer a valid surrogate for the state of an irradiated organism. The live response to a microscopic attack at the cellular level may be compared with that of an individual to a macroscopic attack of the common-or-garden variety. Conscious individuals react and protect themselves in the light of their experience—a learning process that copes with wind and weather, competition with other humans, the search for food and shelter, and more.

The behavior of living cells in response to an attack by ionizing radiation is similar but with three major differences. First, the spectral energy is vastly greater than the feeble energies that bind and regulate the behavior of biological molecules. This imbalance in energy might appear overwhelming. Second, the damage is localized to a few sites by the quantum nature of the energy deposition, other sites being undisturbed. Third, the strategy of attack, that is how the physical science works, never changes and never evolves. This is in stark contrast to an attack by a virus or bacterium for which the energy is quite modest, but the mechanism of the attack can evolve and so be unexpected. In that case, protection is often questionable and needs updating by either evolved immunity or vaccination.

However, there is no vaccine for the effect of a dose of ionizing radiation—and, in fact, none is needed. That is because the mechanism of an attack by radiation never changes, all that biology needed was a "data set" of experiences from which to learn a series of defenses—think artificial intelligence (AI)! The data have been provided by the experience of radiation over millions of years—and they get updated on a daily timescale too.

8.3.2 Background Radiation

Life on the Earth has always existed in an environment of ionizing radiation, and so the need to cope with radiative attacks has always been present. The radiation derives from distant cosmic activity in space and from the current decay of Earth-bound "natural" radioactivity whose origin pre-dates the formation of the Solar system—plus the exposures arising from personal medical treatment.[5] When life began on the Earth some three billion years ago, any dose of radiation from radioactivity would have been somewhat higher than today, but the cosmic flux then is unknown. However, the variation in dose between different geographical locations today is much larger. Naturally occurring radioactivity is due to Uranium-235, Uranium-238, Thorium-232, and Potassium-40, all with exceptionally long lifetimes, have decayed somewhat over billions of years. The average exposure includes significant contributions from radioactivity internal to our bodies as well as external. The mean radiation exposure at sea level in the UK is 2.7 mGy per year,[6] but dose rates as high as 100–200 mGy per year are found in many places in the world, such as the monazite beaches in Brazil [4].

The cosmic radiation flux varies too, increasing where the shielding by the Earth's magnetic field and its atmosphere is reduced—that is at higher magnetic latitude and lower atmospheric pressure. Typical annual exposures in medicine have increased steadily in recent decades—and then there is the therapeutic exposure to radioactive waters at spas that have been fashionable since Roman times. Such treatment is often available on health insurance even where social fear of radiation is prevalent.

8.3.3 Biology, Designed to Maximize Survival

The biology of life has evolved and fashioned itself to survive in the environment where it finds itself. It is popular to refer to a Goldilocks Environment in which the survival of life is optimal—and to suppose that is close to the condition of the Earth today. However, unexpected manifestations of life have been found in extreme conditions suggesting that it is life that matches itself to the environment wherever possible. The recently discovered planets may one day reveal a spectrum of viable Goldilocks conditions that we have not yet appreciated.

---

[5]These are quoted for average diagnostic procedures. Individual therapeutic doses are a thousand times greater for those who receive them. The medical profession is reticent about discussing the figures in front of patients for fear of deterring them from accepting life-saving cancer treatment.

[6]Doses are given in mSv or mGy in the literature sources. The distinction is ignored here.

We observe that life exploits the resilience of multiplicity on two distinct levels. Firstly, the population of each species is composed of many separate but similar individual organisms—if some die, others may live and the species survives. Anyway, all are replaced by fresh copies in the slow regular cycle of sex, birth, and death. Secondly, each organism is composed of many individual cells—if one fails, the design ensures that there is another to take its place. These, too, are regularly replaced, but on a faster cycle.

Oxidation, whether by chemical agents or ionizing radiation, inflicts physical damage at the cellular level. Cells defend themselves, individually, and collectively, using several independent mechanisms.

- Antioxidant resources quench any marauding ROS fragments. A depletion of antioxidants sends a chemical message to unimpaired cells triggering defensive measures.
- An early response to an acute attack triggers a suspension of the cell cycle. This conserves resources and prevents the copying of damaged cells. Unless the attack is contained and this cell maintenance is restarted, cells collectively start to fail leading to acute radiation syndrome (ARS) and thence possible death for the organism as a whole.
- In a damaged cell within an hour or two, enzymes repair any single-strand breaks in the DNA molecules within the nucleus,[7] using the unbroken strand to ensure the genetic code is faithfully reinstated. Double-strand breaks are also repaired but more slowly.
- Triggered by chemical messaging any cells that show signs of damage are killed off, a process called apoptosis.
- Immune system vigilance.

8.3.4 Threshold Mechanism

The net result is illustrated in Fig. 8.3. Instead of the linear response to the stress of the attack arising from the immediate physical attack shown by the dashed line, a net biological response shown by the thick curve describes how the damage for low and moderate stress has been corrected. However, at a certain stress, the damage rises, this is the threshold of lasting damage. This happens because to

[7]The word *nucleus*, as used here, refers to the cell nucleus, not the atomic nucleus.

maintain a large inventory of defensive resources is biologically expensive. The threshold occurs for a stress sufficiently large to exhaust the biological defenses. The biological reaction is a feedback mechanism that protects the stability of the tissue within a certain range, not unlike the action of feedback in electronic and other engineering systems. The LNT account of lasting damage is not compatible with the feedback provided by biology.

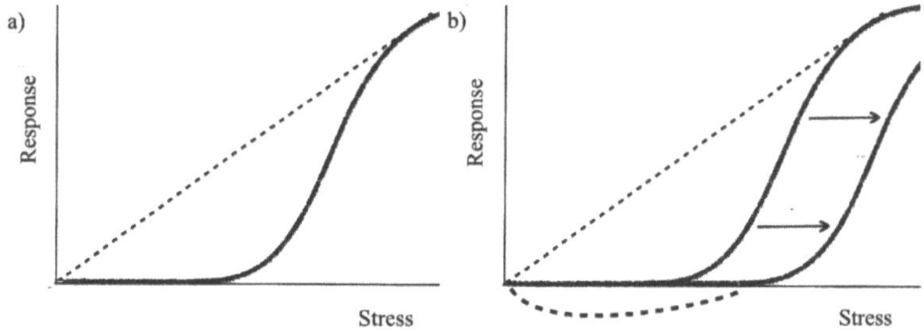

Figure 8.3 (a) The stress-response curve in the presence of stabilizing feedback gives rise to a threshold stress at which the feedback is insufficient to compensate. (b) The stress-response curve changes following an attack, as described in the text.

8.3.5 Adaptation

Following an attack, the inventories of antioxidants and enzymes are replenished—and indeed augmented. In this way, cells in the tissue increase their resilience to a subsequent attack despite the cost of the additional resources required. This simple form of adaptation necessarily changes the curve sketched in Fig. 8.3a. The improved resilience corresponds to an increased threshold with a shift of the solid curve to greater stress levels, as sketched in Fig. 8.3b.

As already discussed, the oxidative damage caused by ionizing radiation and its ROS can also arise from chemical agents unrelated to radiation. The damage from such attacks is made good by many of the same mechanisms and resources as those protecting against radiation. As a result, the adaptive reaction to a radiation dose improves the health outcome for these non-radiative insults, and vice versa. To this extent, exposure to sub-threshold doses of radiation, like regular exercise, can improve health generally. This is called

Hormesis, but giving it a name is not important. It does suggest that a dose of radiation may be beneficial in its effect, depending critically on the dose. And this is true of other agents too. As Paracelsus, physician and botanist (1493–1541), wrote "*Poison is in everything, and nothing is without poison. The dosage makes it either a poison or a remedy*." For this reason, the dose-response curve is sometimes drawn as having a negative response for low doses, as illustrated by the heavy dashed curve in Fig. 8.3b.

8.3.6 Where Mathematics Fails to Work

Such a curve is illustrative at best, but it should not be elevated to the status of a mathematical function. Ionizing radiation is just one of many stresses like mental exertion, diet, and physical exercise. Also, there are many responses too. This description of many curves on many different diagrams is losing the obvious appeal of the original simple mathematical picture. However, the description of adaptation brings other problems.

Normal feedback may be described as a cause-effect relationship, which minimizes, if not cancels, the effect below a certain threshold, as in Fig. 8.3a. However, if the feedback is adaptive, the curve itself moves following the application of stress. So, the feedback modifies itself in the light of experience and depends on the history of past stresses. At its most meaningful, the curve might be defined for constant chronic stress, but in general, the whole description using a mathematical function becomes ephemeral.

Faith in the cultural superiority of mathematics grew from its extraordinarily precise predictive power in engineering and physical science that the world had already come to respect. However, it was gobsmacked at the surprise culmination of the secret Manhattan Project. This has given undeserved credibility to the use of mathematics in forecasting behavior, and thence the outcome, in all manner of applications. The illogical use of mathematical functions is widespread in finance, for instance, where its numerical techiness is seen as sophisticated. The facile use of linear regression is no more than illustrative unless its relevance is backed by mechanism. In market dynamics, a rising price generates reactions that tend to lower it again. Faith in "resistance levels" and trends found by mathematical fitting tend to disappoint.

The unsuitability of physical science for predicting events in biology can be illustrated with a simple story. A marathon race is announced. A physicist and a biologist plan to enter. The physicist considers the enormous energy he will need on the day. How can he be sure to get it? He arranges an energy-rich diet and stays in bed for a month before the race. The biologist is also impressed by the task. For weeks before, the race he trains, setting himself a training routine of running, each day going a little further or a little faster. When the race day comes, they both start off, but after just a mile and a half, an ambulance is heard. There are no prizes for guessing which competitor it comes to collect!

A biological response comprises several mechanisms, which can be trained by adaptation for the task in hand—for ionizing radiation, just as for other tasks, in which we engage. The difference from physical training is that we do not feel the changes that ionizing radiation induces at the cellular level. But then neither are we aware of a similar cellular action induced by vaccination or taking antibiotics. That does not worry us much, assuming we trust the technology.

All life is protected from low and moderate exposure to ionizing radiation. All plants and animals have adapted to the same environment, unconsciously over billions of years, otherwise, life including humans would not be here today. So, only humans are bothered by variations in radiation exposure. Flora and fauna in the Evacuation Zone at Chernobyl are blissfully unaware that, almost without exception, they have benefited from fully paid-up radiological protection. It was only the humans that panicked.

8.3.7 Response Time, Chronic and Acute Threshold

An important question is how long it takes for these protective cellular mechanisms to work. This response time, typically a day or two, is similar to the biological recovery time for other injuries and is linked to the cell cycle which also varies. Within a response time, the effect of any dose accumulates, as envisaged in LNT. In the absence of adaptation, the damage incurred by this integrated dose may trigger permanent damage according to the dose-response curve. Any dose delivered after the response time would not increase the total stress that determines whether the cellular defenses are overwhelmed according to the curve. However, if the curve is altered by adaptation, the shape of the curve is transitory and this description becomes invalid. Adaptation can be stimulated by stress below the threshold for lasting damage—in fact, it continuously monitors the biological resources likely needed to cope with an increased dose.

The lasting damage to an organism caused by a dose of radiation may involve a shortening of life, the incidence of a specific disease such as cancer, or a change in the genetic code that gets passed to later generations. In each case, the threshold for damage by a chronic exposure may be expressed as a dose rate, while that for an acute exposure is a dose. So, they are different in principle, though frequently confused. Naturally, if adaptive mechanisms are active, the threshold for any acute stress depends on the exposure history and is not related to the response to chronic stress. Since exposure histories may vary, caution is needed in any discussion on the damage threshold for an acute dose.

Some response times can be measured in vitro in the laboratory. For example, single-strand DNA breaks are repaired in hours. Another important source of evidence is fractionation, the segmentation of a radiotherapy dose into daily deliveries of 2 Gy to a tumor over 5–6 weeks. A century of experience by oncologists has shown that this usually proves fatal to the cancer cells while nearby healthy tissue usually recovers from receiving 1 Gy per day during the treatment. Of course, it would be cheaper and simpler to deliver a monthly dose of 40 Gy or more in a single treatment, but without the opportunity to recover from the daily dose, the nearby tissue does not survive such treatment. Admittedly, secondary cancers can occur with a small percentage risk and tissue may be burnt but oncologists have a century and more of experience of steering a treatment between these treatable risks and the chance of failing to kill the tumor cells.

A limit defined for safe exposure to ionizing radiation is not the same as the many thresholds that may be found in scientific studies of enduring radiation damage. The latter will vary with experience and individual health characteristics. The former should be a single dose rate, simply described, and cautiously defined to cover the majority of the scientific findings, but not with unprovoked powers of ten that will add, or rather multiply, costs when implemented in regulations. "Simply described" means it should be taught in schools and explained to the public. Politicians, media commentators, and courts of law should understand and respect it. Unfortunately, in the past 70 years, the image of nuclear technology has been damaged by ignorance and fear. The reasons for this mistrust and how it can be overcome are discussed in the next section.

8.4 The Social Response

8.4.1 Objectivity and Perception of Self

There is a qualitative barrier between human perceptions of the outside world and the subjective self, usually veiled in unexpressed uncertainty. The intrusion of science near this barrier causes angst, as did Charles Darwin's work, for example. The acceptance of his thesis left open the question of how variations of human life originated, or of any other life—for there is supposed to be no distinction. A rising interest in eugenics in the first half of the 20th century—and the racism that it so easily encourages—is an attempt to protect the inheritance of self and its values. In the absence of any competing mechanism, there was an expectation among many geneticists that ionizing radiation should be the agent that induces inheritable changes to the germplasm. Notable among these was Hermann Muller for whom this mechanism was self-evident. Indeed, he was awarded the Nobel Prize in Physiology in 1946 for his earlier work on fruit flies, although it did not confirm the mutations that he supposed [5]. Furthermore, any detectable occurrence of inherited genetic changes in humans by ionizing radiation has been essentially excluded by multi-generational studies of the survivors of the 1945 bombing of Hiroshima and Nagasaki [6]. However, this was never explained to the public, or indeed to the wider scientific community. The ghoulish images of life permanently changed by the effect of radiation have persisted for many decades, misleading general scientific and political opinion as well as spicing the plot of horror stories and films. Indeed, for many in society, the responsibility for allowing such irreversible interference with subsequent generations raised sufficient political pressure to halt the Arms Race in the Cold War.

8.4.2 The Placebo and Nocebo Effects

Other sources of social pressure influence reactions to radiation. It is regrettable, one might say, that humans are not like animals. They know too much—and too little. What they do know simply scares them. Safety information is easily misunderstood when passed to others, either by authorities who themselves do not understand or by public discussion that can easily spread panic. It is well-known that the influence of thought on health is problematic, for instance, in assessing the efficacy of drugs and vaccines. Patients who think that they have received treatment when they have not, are apt to show better recovery than those in the population who do not even think they have been treated. This is the Placebo Effect. To overcome it, a blind trial is performed with two groups, one who is treated and one who is not, without them knowing to which group they belong. Ideally, a similar innocence would enable a proper assessment of the effects of ionizing radiation. This is simple with groups of animals. Mice are used in high statistics studies, in particular, to investigate fetal and reproductive sensitivity. For whole-of-life studies, dogs are used because their longevity is better matched to that of humans.

However, there is also a malign counterpart to the Placebo Effect in which a human thinks he has been harmed when he has not. This is called the Nocebo Effect and is evident in primitive societies as a curse or voodoo. But no one is completely immune, and even the most educated are sensitive to the depressing effect of a comment such as "You don't look too good today! Are you alright?" Published accounts describe how genuine suffering, even death, may be induced by suggestion [7].

The inhabitants of the Evacuation Zone at Chernobyl were told "*You have been irradiated,*" and buses were arranged to take them from their homes, permanently and without notice. Not all went, and those who stayed behind survived better as a result. The UN Report of 2006 [8] confirmed widespread mental illness, alcoholism, family break up, and misery among the evacuees.

The lesson was not learned and a similarly disastrous evacuation was hastily arranged following the Fukushima Daiichi accident [9]. Evacuees were told to apply for large sums in compensation. Not only did this add to the supposed cost of the accident, but it also motivated the public to maximize the effect on their lives. No one at all died from the ionizing radiation, while, in contrast, the earthquake and tsunami caused a death toll of some 18,000 with harrowing details that received less media attention [10]. Meanwhile, in their business interest, the organs of modern publicity added to the fearful image of radiation around the world. However, the public already experiences rather intense exposure to ionizing radiation and treats them as acceptable.

8.4.3 Ultraviolet Radiation in Sunshine

Popular attitudes to ultraviolet radiation are calm and relatively informed, even if not always careful. UV is absorbed naturally by exposed tissue, for instance, when sunbathing. The longer wavelengths in the solar spectrum, i.e., the optical and infrared regions, provide the warmth the sunbather seeks. In the atmosphere, in particular, the ozone layer absorbs wavelengths shorter than 280 nm (UVC), but exposure in the range shorter than 315 nm (UVB) is absorbed by the skin and is harmful. Sunscreens and blocks containing high Z elements like zinc and titanium can provide some protection. Otherwise, the radiation kills cells in the skin, which then peel off and is replaced in a few days. But, just as for other kinds of ionizing radiation, adaptation is significant. In the first few days of a vacation in the Sun, extra caution is needed to avoid severe sunburn. Later the skin adapts, the threshold rises and longer periods in the midday Sun become tolerable.

But, as many know their cost, cellular protection and replacement sometimes fail. Such errors, if not caught and neutralized by the immune system, can give rise to cancer, often years later. Although skin cancer is a more significant cause of death than that due to other ranges of ionizing radiation, the public image of exposure to ultraviolet is not a matter of panic. Concern is handled through doctors, pharmacists, and parents so that children learn to trust and enjoy their holidays in the sunshine. Significantly, there is no LNT, no dose-response curve, just a safe exposure, barrier cream, and a sun hat. International advice from a UN committee plays no role as it has come to do for other forms of ionizing radiation. But melanoma skin cancer is serious. Between 2% and 3% of UK residents will be diagnosed with it in their lifetime of which 86% are caused by overexposure to UV. In 2017–2019, 1% of all cancer deaths in the UK were attributed to melanoma [11]. Other causes of cancer listed by Cancer Research UK include smoking, obesity, alcohol, and diet. Notably, apart from UV, ionizing radiation does not make the list [12].

Public policy and safety regulations should be consistent with scientific evidence, but also carry economic needs and public education with them. It is helpful to think of cases where such apparently incompatible requirements were resolved in the past. Such is the regulation of highway safety, today, achieved by policies that are widely accepted, understood, and supported through education. Guided by data on the damage caused in vehicle-pedestrian collisions at different speeds and the likelihood of a pedestrian being on the roadway, regulations on maximum permitted speed are agreed upon, even though it is accepted that additional care is needed for children and old people. These regulations are regularly reviewed and updated following improvements in engineering and the education of drivers and pedestrians. However, research to find a finely honed mathematical cause-and-effect curve to describe accidents is not a priority. As for highway speeds, the limit for radiological exposures should be as high as relatively safe (AHARS)—the qualification 'relatively' meaning that the consequences of a tighter limit would incur greater risks to life in other respects. If the intention is to remove all risk, regardless, the limit would be set as low as reasonably achievable (ALARA), similar to a highway requirement for vehicles to reach their destination only eventually. That would be an application of the so-called Precautionary Principle—a preposterous name given to a counsel of fear and presumed ignorance. For vehicles that was indeed the philosophy in use before 1896 (in the UK) when vehicle speeds were limited to three miles an hour. Why? Because the public was frightened by the idea of huge steam locomotives on the highway. But the regulations were changed when much smaller cars appeared from France and Germany. The economic prospects opened up by the switch were overwhelming, as we now know. A similar transition is to be expected with nuclear power and its regulation, but that depends on repealing the radiological equivalent of the Red Flag Act that required someone to walk in front of a motor car waving a flag—a safety regulation dependent on ALARA.

8.4.4 The International Assessment of Radiological Safety, 1934

Early experiments with ionizing radiation revealed that excess exposure caused inflammation of the skin, like sunburn but more penetrating. The history is well described with references and illustrations by Mould [13]. Radiation therapy as a cure for cancers and many other conditions soon developed. But in the early years, there was little information on radiation-induced cancers, in part, because these generally take some years to develop, but also because ionizing radiation is a rather weak carcinogen. This long latency before disease appears is probably caused by the weakening of the immune system with increasing age.

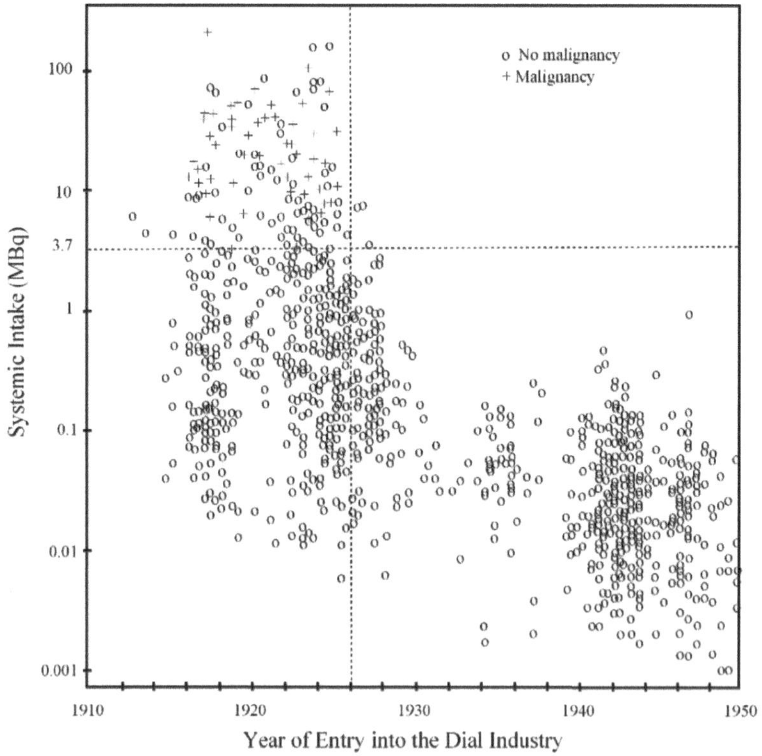

Figure 8.4 Dial painters. From Ref. [14].

An early source of significant data was the experience of the workers, who painted the luminous dials of watches and instruments with radium paint [14]. Before 1926, to get the finest results many of them licked the tip of their brushes. Radium is a calcium-like element and the Radium-226 was absorbed in their bones. With its half-life of 1600 years, this gave them a lifelong internal dose of radiation and a significant likelihood of bone cancer, an otherwise relatively unusual disease. The data are shown in Fig. 8.4. Painters who died of bone cancer are shown as + marks. Of the 191 painters who ingested an activity of more than 3.7 MBq (marked by the horizontal dashed line), 46 died of cancer. Among 1339 painters who ingested less, there were no cases. From 1926 onwards, marked by the dashed line, the practice of licking was discouraged, the doses fell and no further cases of bone cancer were found. The alpha decay energy of Radium-226 is 4.79 MeV and so for a 70 kg person, an activity of 3.7 MBq corresponds to a dose rate of 3.5 mGy per day. This is a measure of a life-long chronic threshold.

International Recommendations 1

INTERNATIONAL RECOMMENDATIONS FOR X-RAY AND RADIUM PROTECTION

REVISED BY THE INTERNATIONAL X-RAY AND RADIUM PROTECTION COMMISSION AT THE FOURTH INTERNATIONAL CONGRESS OF RADIOLOGY, ZÜRICH, JULY 1934.

Members

Dr. R. Ledoux-Lebard (France), Chairman.
Dr. G. W. C. Kaye (National Physical Laboratory, England), Honorary Secretary.
Prof. R. Bär (Switzerland).
Dr. H. Behnken (Physikalisch-Technische Reichsanstalt, Germany).
Dr. R. Sievert (Sweden).
Dr. I. Solomon (Service d'Etalonnage de l'Hôpital St. Antoine, Paris).
Prof. F. Tank (Switzerland).
Dr. L. S. Taylor (National Bureau of Standards, U.S.A.).
Dr. E. Pugno-Vanoni (Italy).

INTERNATIONAL RECOMMENDATIONS

1. The dangers of over exposure to X rays and radium can be avoided by the provision of adequate protection and suitable working conditions. It is the duty of those in charge of X-ray and radium departments to ensure such conditions for their personnel. The known effects to be guarded against are:—

(*a*) Injuries to the superficial tissues.

(*b*) Derangements of internal organs and changes in the blood.

The evidence at present available appears to suggest that under satisfactory working conditions a person in normal health can tolerate exposure to X rays to an extent of about 0·2 international röntgens (r) per day. On the basis of continuous irradiation during a working day of seven hours, this figure corresponds to a dosage rate of 10^{-5} r per second. The protective values given in these recommendations are generally in harmony with this figure under average conditions. No similar tolerance dose is at present available in the case of radium gamma rays.

Figure 8.5 The text of the 1934 guidance on radiation tolerance. From Ref. [15].

The experience of the 1920s and early 1930s led in 1934 to an agreement on a safe dose rate. The text agreed by the International X-ray and Radium Protection Commission, the forerunner of the International Commission for Radiological Protection (ICRP), is shown in Fig. 8.5. The agreed general threshold was set at 0.2 roentgen per day, equivalent to 2 mGy per day in modern units, close to the chronic threshold calculated from the Dial Painter data.

But 1934 is nearly a century ago. Is that threshold still valid? Today, not only are there far better data but many of the mechanisms of the biological response are understood. The members of that 1934 Committee included Rolf Sievert and Lauriston Taylor, doyen of radiation physicists and chairman of US NCRP for 48 years. Nearly 50 years later, Taylor spoke of the persistent validity of that threshold when he delivered the Sievert Lecture at the Fifth International Congress of the Radiation Protection Association. He said: "*Today we know about all we need to know for adequate protection against ionizing radiation.*" On page 856: "*No one has been identifiably injured by radiation while working within the first numerical standard set by NCRP and the ICRP in 1934*" [16]. Toward the end of this prescient article, he said "*The press in dealing with our protection problems lends favor to charlatans—individuals who know how to make headlines and become known to the public as 'the authorities'.*" He is saying that an effective safety regime needs to be based on science and also be shared effectively with society at large. As he said it was misrepresented in 1980, and that is no less true today.

Members of the public accept the personal health benefits of the clinical doses given for cancer therapy. Every member of the public has a friend or relative who has benefited from high doses of radiation, even if they have not themselves. These are compared with the recommendations of 1934 in Fig. 8.6 as the area of circles. The outer red circle represents the therapy dose delivered to a tumor. At about 2 Gy per day for 20 days per month kills cells. The yellow circle corresponds to a dose received by healthy tissue close to the tumor, which usually recovers after treatment. The green circle, about 200 times smaller, corresponds to the limit set in 1934. With this sturdy factor, it is not surprising that there is no evidence to suggest damage at a lesser exposure, either in a health clinic or in the environment—even among the survivors of Hiroshima and Nagasaki.

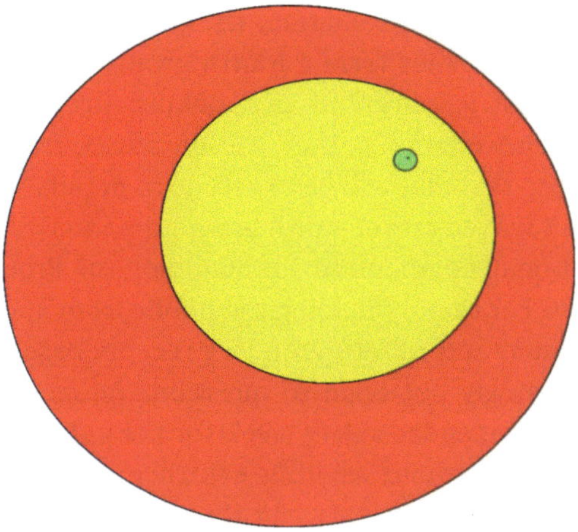

Figure 8.6 Circles with areas corresponding to radiation dose rates.

If media and politicians' influence would engage with the evidence responsibly, the image of nuclear technology that shines in health would shine in environmental activity too.

8.5 Conclusions

Today, society includes groups of people with seemingly disparate views. A task for the future of humanity, more important even than the development of new sources of energy, is to get these groups to engage with one another. It is a matter of education and discussion.

One group has a professional grasp of the physics and engineering of nuclear technology, but no real confidence in biology. A second group is health care professionals. Their first concern is the health of their patients and they are reluctant to engage in any discussion likely to upset the willingness of their patients to accept treatment. Being less familiar with the physics of nuclear and its radiation, many are in awe of its extreme energy. Most members of the general public from a third group have never really been told about the science. At school, teaching tip-toes around the "controversial" bits as quickly as possible. Instead, they have views accumulated from media reports that alarm with inherited nuclear propaganda dating from the Cold War. For them, nuclear technology is political, unnatural, and man-made. They believe the danger of nuclear war is dominated by the deadly effects of radiation, its spread, and its persistence. The political authorities form a fourth group whose priorities are the avoidance of liability and civil disturbance. Since they have no personal understanding, they call on advice from professional experts, hoping that that will be to accede to popular demands.

The result was to create a fifth group, the international experts, the International Commission for Radiological Protection (ICRP) under the UN. For them, shielding the public from nuclear radiation is a commitment and ALARA with its precepts based on LNT is an ideology, seemingly not open to question. To satisfy the political group, the recommended safety levels for the public were tightened by a factor of 700 without scientific evidence.

The stasis of opinion between these groups remained frozen by ignorance and inertia from the 1950s until the early years of the new millennium. The inertia comes largely from the desire for job security that obstructs change. Young people selecting a career and employer are the major drivers of change. Today, they can see how the status quo obstructs the provision of cheap nuclear energy. With the wholesale reduction in the use of fossil fuels and the evident inadequacy of wind and solar, the need for a widespread reconsideration of the cultural aversion to nuclear technology is essential. This aversion increases the costs of nuclear power but has no basis in natural science, as this chapter has shown.

Two generations of education reform and public information are now required, worldwide, and across political persuasions.

References

1. Allison W. *Fundamental Physics for Probing and Imaging.* ISBN 9780199203888. Oxford University Press, 2006. https://global.oup.com/academic/product/fundamental-physics-for-probing-and-imaging-9780199203888
2. Harrison J, Leggett R, Lloyd D, Phipps A, Scott B. Polonium-210 as a poison. *J Radiol Prot.* 2007, 27(1), 17–40. https://www.ncbi.nlm.nih.gov/pubmed/17341802/
3. *The Drama of Plutonium,* Nuclear Energy International https://www.neimagazine.com/opinion/opinionthe-drama-of-plutonium
4. Richel T. *No More Radiophobia!* A professionally made video. 2020. https://youtu.be/JpcUCo0ebNA

5. Calabrese EJ. Confirmation that Hermann Muller was dishonest in his Nobel Prize Lecture. *Arch Arch Toxicol.* 2023, 97, 2999–3003. https://doi.org/10.1007/s002
6. Nakamura N. Genetic effects of radiation in atomic-bomb survivors and their children: past, present and future. *Radiat Res.* 2006, 47 (Suppl. B), B67–B73. Available at https://doi.org/10.1269/jrr.47.B67.
7. Pilcher H. *The Science of Voodoo: When The Mind Attacks The Body.* 2009. https://www.newscientist.com/article/mg20227081-100-the-science-of-voodoo-when-mind-attacks-body/ also https://possiblemind.co.uk/voodoo-when-mind-attacks-body/
8. WHO. *Report of the UN Chernobyl Forum Expert Group "Health".* 2006. https://iris.who.int/bitstream/handle/10665/43447/9241594179_eng.pdf
9. Allison W. Viewpoint: We should stop running away from radiation. 2011. https://philpapers.org/asearch.pl?pub=3132; https://www.bbc.co.uk/news/world-12860842
10. Parry RL. *Ghosts of the Tsunami: Death and Life in Japan.* ISBN-:9781911214 Jonathan Cape, 2017.
11. *Melanoma Skin Cancer Risk*, Cancer Research UK. https://www.cancerresearchuk.org/health-professional/cancer-statistics/statistics-by-cancer-type/melanoma-skin-cancer/risk-factors#heading-Zero
12. *Causes of Cancer and Reducing Your Risk*, Cancer Research UK. https://www.cancerresearchuk.org/about-cancer/causes-of-cancer
13. Mould RE. *A Century of X-Rays and Radioactivity in Medicine.* London: Institute of Physics Publishing, 1993.
14. Rowland RE. *Radium Dial Painters – What Happened to Them?* 2004. www.rerowland.com/Dial_Painters.pdf
15. *International Recommendations.* 1934, published by ICRP. https://www.icrp.org/images/1934.JPG
16. Taylor LS. Some non-scientific influences on radiation protection standards and practice. The 1980 Sievert Lecture, *Health Physics.* 1980, 39(6), 851–74. https://pubmed.ncbi.nlm.nih.gov/7204045/

Chapter 9

Transport of Radioactive Materials

Franco Cioce
Curator of Museum of Radioactivity, Radiation Protection Expert – Dangerous Goods Safety Adviser
fcioce@gmail.com

Transportation, one of the activities always present in every operational field, is an independent activity that deserves proper protection and consideration. It is held within many different sites, from inhabited centers to crowded roads used by ordinary citizens who know nothing of what is being transported.

Radioactive materials used in industry, agriculture, medicine, and other fields also fall within the case of transport. Every year, worldwide, over 20 million shipments are made within countries and across borders.

There are also radioactive sources that must be transported to specialized centers and disposed of.

In a confined structure, such as a hospital or a manufacturing company, the systems and safety measures, as well as the control levels, make much easier the safe storage and conservation of radioactive sources.

Radioactivity in Life Sciences
Edited by Maria Letizia Terranova

ISBN 978-981-5129-67-0 (Hardcover), 978-1-003-63654-0 (eBook)
www.jennystanford.com

Conversely during transport, especially on road (road mode), the operational variables multiply and necessarily involve people cars that pass alongside the vehicle carrying the radioactive material (Fig. 9.1).

In such cases, even a minimal accident such as a simple rear-end collision could lead to a traffic stop precisely because of the fear generated by the mandatory warning signs that the vehicle must show during transport.

Precisely to address and resolve these aspects, the International Atomic Energy Agency (IAEA) has published a regulation [1], which indicates the safety criteria to be implemented, from the classification of what can be transported up to the choice of the ideal container and of the proper signaling.

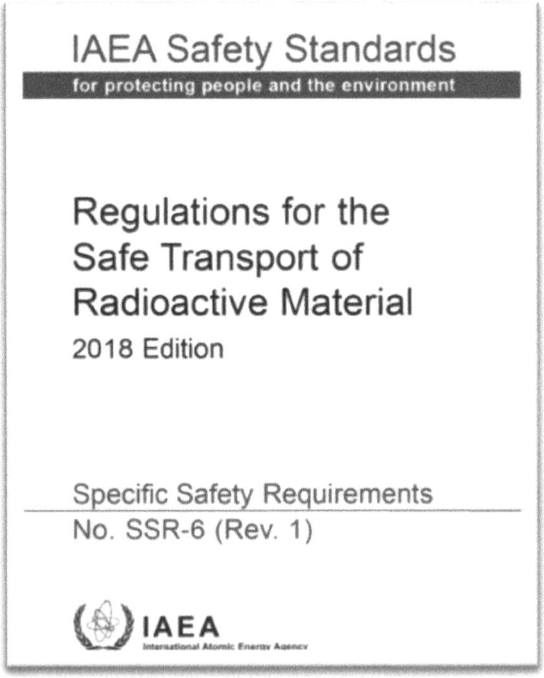

Figure 9.1 IAEA 2018 Regulations for the Safe Transport of Radioactive Material.

The United Nations adopted the technical and scientific indications proposed by the IAEA and included the safety criteria in the ADR regulation (regulation for the safe road transport of dangerous goods) modeling and expanding them on "urban" realities (parking of vehicles, safety equipment, information to the competent authorities, etc.) [2] (Fig. 9.2).

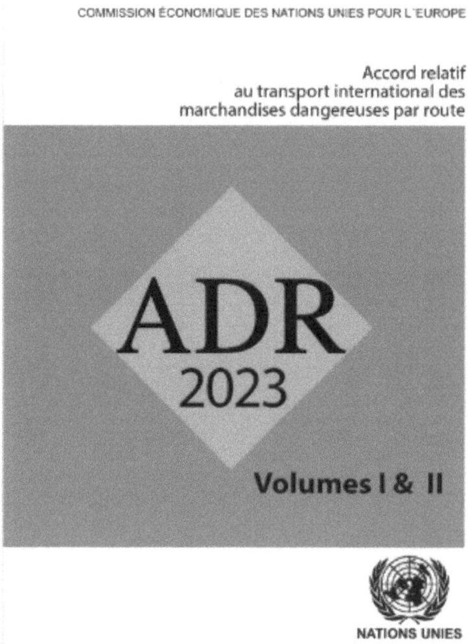

Figure 9.2 ADR 2023 Regulations.

We are all well aware that there is transport which, depending on the nature, size, or dangerousness of the material, is escorted by technical services or law enforcement to guarantee the security of the delicate transport phase and the safety of customers on the road.

But this procedure is carried out in a small percentage compared to the whole world market and is not applied for the small radioactive sources for industry, healthcare, and to a lesser extent, research, which constitute the majority of radioactive transport and are carried out using normal vans.

Therefore, the main impositions addressed to the shipping of this type of radioactive material are those of using only containers meeting the safety requirements or even "approved" by the authorities who certify the ability to withstand the most serious incidents.

Such containers (called "type B") can accommodate only specific radioactive elements with well-defined activities (quantities), have a limited time validity of 7 years, and must subsequently be renewed in order to continue their use [3] (Fig. 9.3).

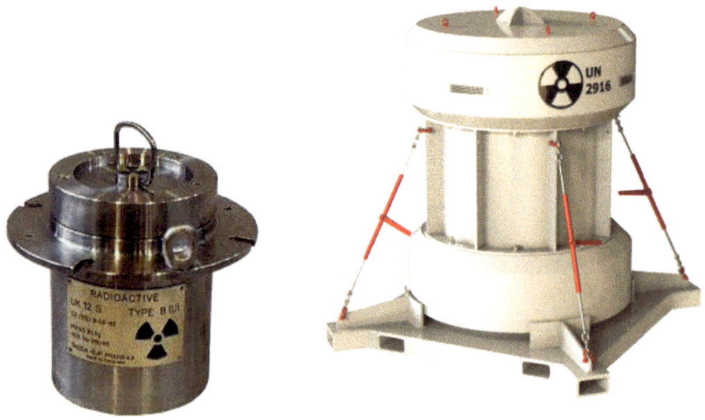

Figure 9.3 Type B containers for transport of radioactive materials.

The containers must have undergone several resistance tests, like immersion in water, exposure to fire, falling from different heights, impact with a pointed object of a defined weight, etc. All this is to certify that the container is also resistant to a variety of accidental stresses.

From the first edition of the IAEA regulation (1961), which established the safety criteria for containers, up to the latest edition of 2018, updated to the activities carried out with the various known radionuclides, the application of the IAEA has allowed the transport of radioactive materials to be carried out with high levels of safety and protection from radiation.

Proof of this is that in over 60 years of transport around the world, no significant events have ever been recorded in terms of exposure of workers or the population or environmental damages.

To give a "dimension" to the safety criteria adopted, one must consider that to transport a small source (a few grams) of iridium used in the health sector for "brachytherapy," a container of almost 30 kg must be used, precisely to limit as much as possible the radiation exposure of the personnel handling these items [4] (Fig. 9.4).

The much heavier container is needed for the transport of more "dangerous" radioactive materials.

In the case of the 60-Co, used in industrial centers to ensure sterilization or a drastic reduction of the bacterial load on many objects for medical and also daily use, containers with a maximum capacity of 10 kg of cobalt can weigh from 4500 to 6000 kg (Fig. 9.5).

It is well-known that radiations have the ability to pass through large thicknesses of material including lead and concrete. Obviously, this does not apply to any radioactive emission, but only to radiations emitted from some radionuclides.

The radiation emitted by some nuclides can be stopped by a thin paper sheet (alpha radiations) while others X or gamma radiations are able to cross up to 100 cm of concrete.

Therefore, the greater the crossing capacity and intensity of the radioactive emission, the thicker the container walls needed to provide effective shielding.

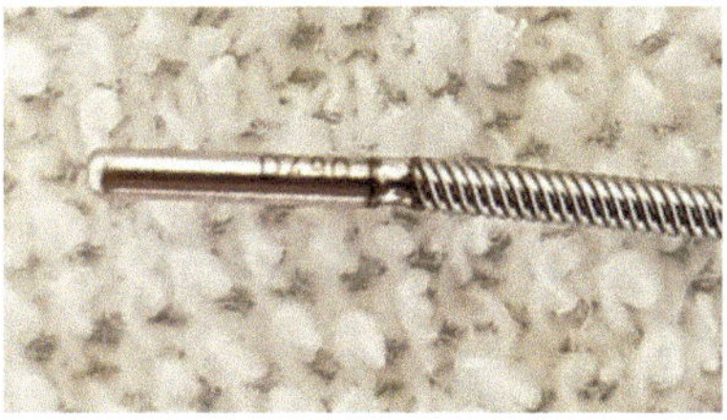

(a)

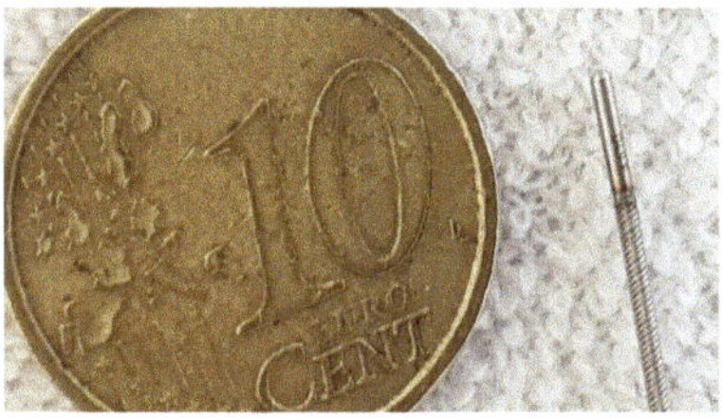

(b)

Figure 9.4 (a) Source of radioactive Ir192 used for per brachytherapy. (b) Indication of the size of the Ir192 source.

For the most penetrating radiations, such as gamma rays, thick-wall containers will never be able to completely stop the radiation emitted from the enclosed radionuclides.

Rather, the thickness and therefore the weight of the container could be increased, but this would then affect the transport and handling capacity. In other words, such packaging would not be able to be transported. Therefore, the international regulations are based on the "acceptability" of the minimum doses emerging from the containers.

The active and passive safety precautions, to which should be added responsible and adequate behaviors, contribute to ensuring transport safety not only for the workers but also for the population [5].

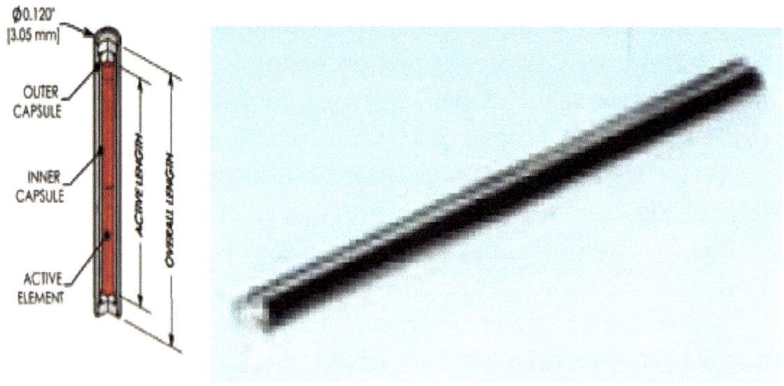

(a)

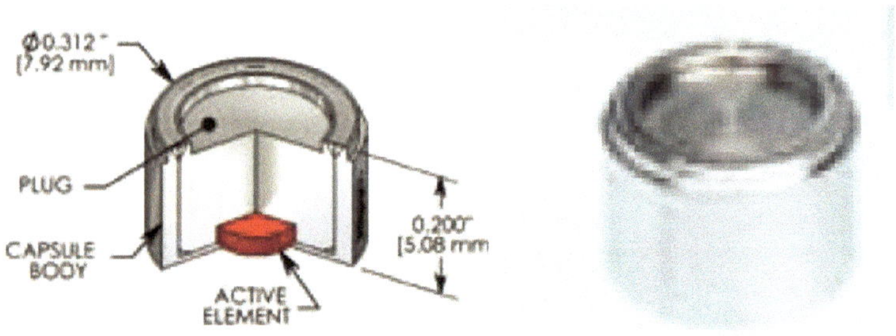

(b)

Figure 9.5 (a) A rod of 60-Co. (b) A capsule containing Cs137.

In this regard, transport safety is addressed not only with adequate transport containers but also with specific training that the driving staff must possess.

Many countries in the world that apply the ADR regulation require drivers of vehicles carrying dangerous goods to follow a 15-day course and submit them to a written examination to demonstrate knowledge of the regulation.

To transport radioactive materials, it is necessary to pass an additional examination precisely because of the specificity of the dangers of this commodity.

The Professional Training Certificate (better known as "ADR license") obtained after the 15-day course and the final examination on "radioactive materials" must be renewed every five years, to guarantee the knowledge of the continuous upgrading of the ADR regulation (which, in turn, is updated every two years).

Obviously, the technical and legislative rules that regulate the safety of transport of radioactive sources take into account, the many existing realities, often not well-known or not considered by many. Examples are all those objects or food that contain radioactive nuclides by nature, without anyone having "introduced" radioactivity inside them. Humanity has always lived with these objects/foods that never caused health troubles.

Think of bananas or nuts or many legumes that contain the naturally radioactive K40 potassium nuclide. And think also of the beverage par excellence, the water springing from the ground and rocks, carrying with it invisible and microscopic quantities of radioactive elements, including uranium and thorium.

Considering that we have always drunk and will continue to drink these waters without causing any damage to our health, the transport of these items does not fall under ADR rules.

However, despite all the taken precautions, sometimes newspapers and media report that containers with radioactive sources inside have been stolen or lost. In these cases, it is necessary to analyze, even with the help of experts, the veracity of reported news and the real danger to which the population can be exposed.

Looking at the IAEA website that reports and describes all the instances of thefts of radioactive sources, one notes that the sad record for such crimes has been reached by Mexico between 2013 and 2017.

In all these cases, it turned out that thefts were not aimed directly at the radioactive material (which we have seen to be of minimal size and weight) but at the metal container.

In effect, thieves knew nothing of the contents, or were not interested in them, but were attracted by the considerable mass of the container, which have always been found at illegal resellers of materials and scrap metals.

The safety rules in some cases do not seem to be fully adequate to avoid accidents, as in the recent loss that occurred in Australia in January 2023.

As described by the media, a source of cesium (Cs137) would have leaked from an instrument during a 1400 km transportation and would have fallen on the ground through a small hole in the loading platform of the vehicle. The radioactive source in question was found a few days later without causing damage to the population or the environment. Unfortunately, human errors affect 90% of cases and the correct, constant, and in-depth training of the operators in the presence of well-detailed and well-understood procedures is what can make the difference. Such an accident, regardless of the description offered by the media, must be taken as an example to improve more and more the safety requirements for the transport of dangerous items, and in particular, radioactive ones.

Radioactivity, in people who are not familiar with this topic, generates distrust and fear not only because it is usually associated with dramatic events (atomic bombs, nuclear accidents, etc.) but also because of the peculiar characteristics of nuclear radiation, they cannot be seen, sensed, smell, or in general perceived if not through specific instruments.

Fortunately, the efforts of professionals and institutions in the sector are entirely aimed at the safety of populations, workers, and the environment.

As for many human activities, especially the ones that can create dangers to people's health and security; also in the case of the transport of equipment or substances that produce ionizing radiation, the critical aspects are dealt with in advance.

Nothing is left to chance, and to achieve the required levels of safety, the following points are often taken into consideration:

- Road routes (great mileage roads (motorways) are absolutely favored, trying to avoid road tunnels and limiting as much as possible the crossing of city streets),
- transit times of the vehicle,
- weather conditions foreseen during the route,
- traffic conditions according to travel times,
- the driving hours of the staff, avoiding as far as possible the sleeping of the drivers inside the laden vehicle, and
- the dangerousness of the transported material.

It may therefore happen to many of us to travel along a public road and come across a vehicle (van or truck) that displays orange rectangular panels in front and behind the vehicle and further panels behind and on the sides of the vehicle, with the well-known radiation symbol (Fig. 9.6 a and b).

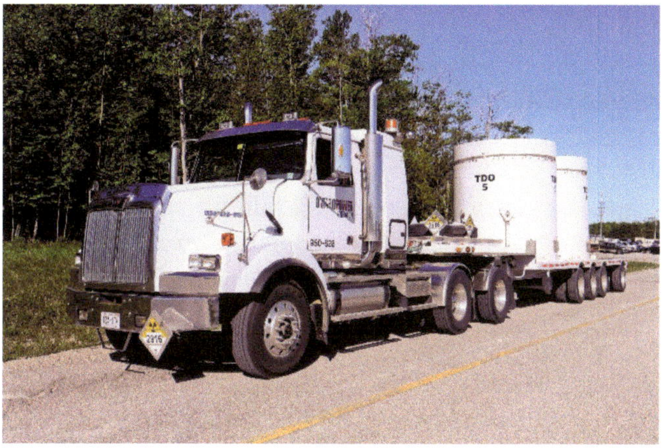

(a)

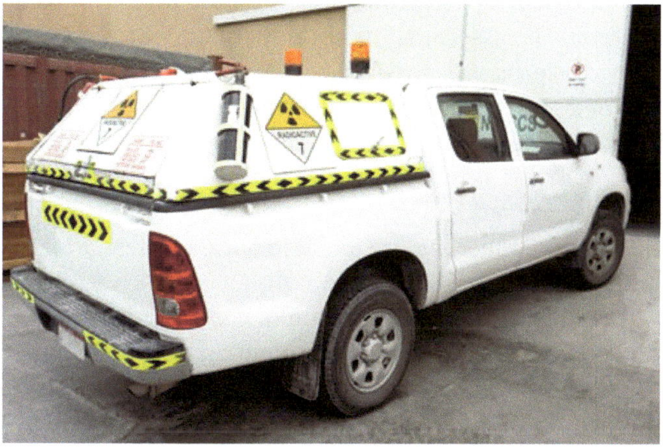

(b)

Figure 9.6 (a) Tractor-trailer for the transport of radioactive sources. (b) Pickup for the transport of small radioactive sources.

The message transmitted through these panels, mandatory in all countries according to IAEA indications, is that the vehicle is carrying radioactive material with values of activity and dose rate (the dose evaluated over an hour of exposure) requiring attention in order to ensure the safety of the population and workers.

As a rule, containers anchored to the loading platform of the vehicle are placed toward the bottom of the platform itself, at a considerable distance from the drivers, so that the emerging dose that can reach the driver's cab is as low as possible.

Even if the dose rate on the rear walls of the vehicle may have higher values than those found in the driver's cab, it must be considered that the exposures of people passing in close proximity to the vehicle are absolutely different from the exposures of the drivers.

These last remain indeed in the cab for the whole time of the journey (and sometimes even during the break, which they must compulsorily observe after a certain period of driving), while the motorists pass by for a few seconds.

We pointed out above that the radioactivity can be found everywhere. Therefore, the many rules that exist for the safe transport of radioactive materials must be applied to everything that has to be transported. Obviously not.

The problem arises from the fact that every time the term "radioactive" is associated with something, the first emotional reaction concerns the possible harm to health. This can mislead uninformed individuals into believing that complete safety is achieved only when there is no radioactivity at all.

However, this is not the case. Radioactivity equal to zero is almost non-existent and radiation emissions, even if minimal and absolutely not dangerous, are found in our daily lives, from food to a lot of items.

It must be noted that a liter of milk has an activity of about 100 Bq (Becquerel: activity unit corresponding to one disintegration/sec), a liter of water can reach 50 Bq, a banana 20 Bq, and a 10 kg block of marble 10,000 Bq. It all depends on the dose.

Paracelsus (1493–1541), a doctor and alchemist accused of having administered poisonous substances to his patients, responded to the slanders claiming that "*Omnia venenum sunt: nec sine veneno quicquam existit. Dosis sola facit, ut venenum non fit.*" (Everything is poison, and nothing exists without poison. Only the dose prevents the poison from taking effect).

A professor at the Enrico Fermi Nuclear Studies Center in Milan Italy (CESNEF) asserted that if it was forbidden to transport any radioactive material without being authorized, then it would also be a crime to carry a passenger in one's car. The reason for this paradoxical statement is determined by the fact that radioactivity does not stop outside our bodies.

A human weighing approximately 70 kg has an activity of about 8000 Bq, of which 5000 Bq, due to the radioactive decay of the "potassium-40" (K40) naturally contained in our bones. In short, radioactivity equal to zero does not exist!

National and international standards are well aware of this, and there are limit values of both total activity (Bq) and specific activity (Bq/g) below which "radioactivity can be neglected."

Also, the ADR regulation for the road transport of "Dangerous Goods" provides exemptions in the case of radioactive materials, that can be freely transported if the indicated specific activity limits (in Bq/g) and total activity limits (in Bq) are not exceeded. Below the values indicated by ADR, the materials are not considered radioactive, therefore the transport phase is not regulated in any way, and there are no obligations regarding labels, containers, equipment, or permits of any kind. Transport in these conditions is absolutely free.

However, the ADR regulation lists further particular cases, regardless of the activity and concentration values, in which the provisions of the same regulation do not apply.

These cases are as follows:

(a) Radioactive material is an integral part of the means of transport.

(b) Radioactive material is moved within an establishment where all the appropriate safety regulations are in operation and where the movement does not involve public roads or railways.

(c) Radioactive material implanted or incorporated into a person or live animal for diagnostic or therapeutic purposes.

(d) Radioactive material that is found in or on the body of a person who is to be transported for medical treatment after accidentally or deliberately absorbing radioactive material or after being contaminated.

(e) Radioactive material contained in consumer products that have received approval from a regulatory body is sold to the final consumer.

(f) Natural materials and minerals containing naturally occurring radionuclides (e.g., tuff bricks or granite and marble).
(g) Non-radioactive solid objects for which the quantities of radioactive materials present on any surface do not exceed the limit indicated in the definition of "contamination."

The same criteria of maximum safety are applied to the radioactive waste.

Unlike the case of non-radioactive dangerous goods, for which the conditions for disposal of waste are different from those of the raw materials, in the case of waste containing radioactive elements, the disposal conditions are in no way different from those established for the radioactive sources in use.

Whereas, the radioactive waste must be observed and strictly applied the criteria for the safety of the population, workers, and environment indicated in the legislative provisions of each country, for their shipment and transport reference must be made only to the specific criteria of the ADR regulation.

The IAEA, which represents one of the many organizations managed by the ONU, requires in an ever more detailed and pressing way that safety be guaranteed, with absolute priority, by all the involved operators.

It is to be noted that in the first edition of this technical regulation the word "waste" appeared only once; for example, in the last edition of 2018, we found it 9 times, mainly associated with "committees" or with the generic safety criteria to be implemented for transport of radioactive material or waste.

This procedure, which deviates from the common approach for the disposal of hazardous and non-hazardous special waste, makes it evident that the management of radioactive waste requires systems of high safety and recognized professional competence.

Whereas for conventional waste, an analytical certificate can help specify contaminants and their concentrations, and consequently outline the danger codes to be reported on the transport document, with radioactive waste, the classification method needs to be changed.

The definition of radioactive waste is as follows:

"Radioactive waste: Any radioactive material in gaseous, liquid, or solid form, even if contained in equipment or devices in general, for which no recycling or further use is foreseen or taken into consideration by

the authority regulator or by a legal or natural person whose decision is accepted by the competent regulatory authority and is regulated as radioactive waste by the competent regulatory authority."

The disposal of radioactive waste is defined as: "*The placing of radioactive waste or spent fuel, in an appropriate manner, in an authorized facility with no intention of subsequently recovering it."*

The IAEA glossary of 2022 [6] is slightly less generic, it refers to a minimal concept of "exemption":

"*For legal and regulatory purposes, material for which no further use is foreseen that contains, or is contaminated with, radionuclides at activity concentrations greater than clearance levels as established by the regulatory body."*

Moreover, in observance of the legislative provisions and authorizations, it is very important to establish whether it is really a disposal rather than a transfer for other reasons.

For example, the need to proceed with a replacement or disposal of the 555 MBq Ni63 source contained in an electron capture detector (ECD) of a common gas chromatograph must be assessed also on the basis of the legal status of the "receiver."

If one intends to proceed with "disposal," then it is necessary to ascertain through the acquisition of documents that the receiving enterprise to which the source is destined, is the entity authorized to operate the reception and disposal of radioactive waste.

In this case, the documentation that will accompany the component to be eliminated must comply with the requirements of the same enterprise that will receive it and must be supplemented by the information required by the ADR regulation.

Otherwise, it will be possible to opt for the "replacement," a possibility always provided by a contractual agreement already established with the supplying enterprise, due to some radioactive sources being foreseen a reuse and to the long life of the radionuclide.

In the latter case, the accompanying documentation will only be that expressly provided for by the ADR regulation and by the law of the country where the transport takes place (transport document).

Within the EU Community, it is necessary to possess the document known as the "EURATOM 1493/93 form" which contains statements by the competent authorities regarding the possibility of receiving that radioactive source or that waste [7]. It is therefore quite intuitive that the ADR regulation is indifferent to regulating the shipping waste or material other than waste. Indeed, it is not even necessary to indicate its nature on the transport document.

If for special waste, thanks to what has been indicated above, it is possible to limit the evaluation investigation to the pertinent hazard class or classes by attributing the worst degree of danger (very dangerous), for radioactive waste this is not possible. It is essential to know in advance:

- the radionuclide,
- its activity at a certain reference date,
- its physical form,
- if in a special form or not,
- if it is a fissile radionuclide,
- the transport category, etc.

The mere fact of making the Geiger counter "ring" is not a sufficient condition to consider when shipping radioactive waste.

In the not improbable case of a mixture of radionuclides, the indications of the ADR regulation itself must therefore be taken into account when calculating the limit values.

Basically, it is necessary to evaluate the fraction of each radionuclide that makes up the mixture and to relate it to the limits that will have to be calculated ex novo.

A package containing radioactive materials can be classified as an exempt package (i.e., the carrier is subjected to less administrative obligations) provided that:

- the radiation intensity at any point on the external surface does not exceed 5 μSv/h;
- the package retains its contents under normal conditions of transport;
- the package bears the indication "RADIOACTIVE" on an internal surface, so as to indicate the presence of radioactive material at the opening of the package, or on the external surface if it is impossible to mark an internal surface;
- or for items too small to bear the marking "RADIOACTIVE," provided that they are transported in a package bearing the indication "RADIOACTIVE" on its inner surface, such that the warning of the presence of radioactive material is visible when the package is opened.

As a whole, in order to transport any object or substance presenting the phenomenon of radioactivity, it is necessary to comply with and fully respect the conditions of absolute safety stated by the operating regulations, in order to guarantee the health of workers and of the population [8].

References

1. IAEA Safety Standards Series No. SSR-6 (Rev.1) – *Specific Safety Requirements, Regulations for the Safe Transport of Radioactive Material*, Edition 2018, STI/PUB/1798 ¦ 978-92-0-107917-6.
2. *Agreement Concerning the International Carriage of Dangerous Goods by Road (ADR), 2023*, ECE/TRANS/326 - ISBN: 978-92-1-139211-1 (English).
3. IAEA Safety Standards Series No. SSG-66 - *Specific Safety Guide - Format and Content of the Package Design Safety Report for the Transport of Radioactive Material*, 2022, STI/PUB/1980 ¦ 978-92-0-141321-5.
4. Franco Cioce - *Classificazione, spedizione e trasporto su strada di materiale radioattivo - Ars Edizioni Informatiche*, 2021, EAN: 9788889260890 - ISBN: 8889260890 - Data di Pubblicazione.
5. IAEA Safety Standards Series No. SSG-26 (Rev. 1) - *Specific Safety Guide - Advisory Material for the IAEA Regulations for the Safe Transport of Radioactive Material*, 2018 Edition, 2022, STI/PUB/1953 - 978-92-0-119021-5.
6. IAEA Nuclear Safety and Security Glossary - *Terminology Used in Nuclear Safety, Nuclear Security - Radiation Protection and Emergency Preparedness and Response*, 2022, (Interim Edition).
7. Regolamento (Euratom) n. 1493/93 del Consiglio, *dell'8 giugno 1993, sulle spedizioni di sostanze radioattive tra gli Stati membri*, 148, 1993, p. 1. ELI: http://data.europa.eu/eli/reg/1993/1493/oj).
8. IAEA Safety Standards Series No. SSG-65 - *Specific Safety Guides – Preparedness and Response for a Nuclear or Radiological Emergency Involving the Transport of Radioactive Material*, 2022, English STI/PUB/1960 ¦ 978-92-0-127521-9.

Index